Quick Reference to Triage

SECOND EDITION

D0619255

Valerie G. A. Grossman, BSN, RN, CEN

Nursing Director for Acute Services
ViaHealth of Wayne:
Newark-Wayne Community Hospital
Newark, New York

Consultant
Triage First, Inc.
Asheville, North Carolina

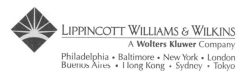

LIPPINCOTT WILLIAMS & WILKINS
A **Wolters Kluwer** Company
Philadelphia • Baltimore • New York • London
Buenos Aires • Hong Kong • Sydney • Tokyo

Acquisitions Editor: Alan Sorkowitz
Editorial Assistant: Megan Klim
Senior Production Editor: Debra Schiff
Senior Production Manager: Helen Ewan
Managing Editor / Production: Erika Kors
Art Director: Brett MacNaughton
Manufacturing Manager: William Alberti
Indexer: Ellen Brennan
Compositor: TechBooks
Printer: RR Donnelly-Crawfordsville

2nd Edition

9 8 7 6 5 4 3 2 1

Library of Congress Cataloging-in-Publication Data

Grossman, Valerie G. A.
   Quick reference to triage / Valerie G.A. Grossman; consultant, Triage First, Asheville, North Carolina.—2nd ed.
      p. cm.
   Includes bibliographical references and index.
   ISBN 0-7817-4022-3
      1. Triage—Handbooks, manuals, etc. I. Title.

RC86.8.G76 2003
616.02′5—dc21   2002040613

   Care has been taken to confirm the accuracy of the information presented and to describe generally accepted practices. However, the author, editors, and publisher are not responsible for errors or omissions or for any consequences from application of the information in this book and make no warranty, express or implied, with respect to the content of the publication.

   The author, editors, and publisher have exerted every effort to ensure that drug selection and dosage set forth in this text are in accordance with the current recommendations and practice at the time of publication. However, in view of ongoing research, changes in government regulations, and the constant flow of information relating to drug therapy and drug reactions, the reader is urged to check the package insert for each drug for any change in indications and dosage and for added warnings and precautions This is particularly important when the recommended agent is a new or infrequently employed drug.

   Some drugs and medical devices presented in this publication have Food and Drug Administration (FDA) clearance for limited use in restricted research settings. It is the responsibility of the health care provider to ascertain the FDA status of each drug or device planned for use in his or her clinical practice.

LWW.com

Dedication

To my husband, Alan

To my children, Nicole and Sarah

To my parents, Marie and John

REVIEWERS *of the Second Edition*

Susan Barnason, PhD, RN
Associate Professor
College of Nursing
University of Nebraska Medical Center
Omaha, Nebraska

Laura A. Bouwens, RN, BSN
Nursing Project Coordinator
ViaHealth of Wayne
Newark, New York

Helen L. Breton, RNC, CEN
Advice Nurse
Southern California Permanente Medical Group
Los Angeles, California

Julie Briggs, RN, BSN, MHA
Director of Emergency and Critical Care
   Services
Good Samaritan Hospital
Puyallup, Washington

Luanne Burcham, RN, BS, ONC
Clinical Manager
Illinois Bone and Joint Institute
Glenview, Illinois

Shelley Cohen, RN, BS, CEN
Educator and Consultant
Health Resources Unlimited
Springfield, Tennessee

Karen L. Dick, RN, PhD, GNP
Assistant Professor
College of Nursing and Health Sciences
University of Massachusetts
Boston, Massachusetts

Angela Falletti, RN
Healthcare Consultant
First Consulting Group
Chantilly, Virginia

Reneé Holleran, RN, PhD, CEN, CCRN, CFRN
Chief Flight Nurse
University Air Care
University Hospital
Cincinnati, Ohio

Elaine Keavney, BSN, RN, CEN
Staff Educator
Good Samaritan Hospital
Puyallup, Washington

Neal L. McGregor, PhD
Professor of Religion and Business
Graceland College
Lamoni, Iowa

Michael S. McNair
Gang & Safety Educator
Triage First, Inc.
Asheville, North Carolina

Rebecca S. McNair, RN, CEN
President
Triage First, Inc.
Asheville, North Carolina

Louise Nelson, BS, RN
Staff Nurse
Optum Nurseline
McLean, Virginia

Sharon Scott, RN, BS
Director of Ambulatory Referral Services
JPS Health Network
Fort Worth, Texas

Patty C. Seneski, RN, ENP, SART, CCAP
Pre-Hospital Manager
Desert Samaritan Medical Center
Mesa, Arizona

Cheryl Sheridan, RN, BS
Director of Acute Services/Behavioral Health
  Network
ViaHealth: Rochester General Hospital
Rochester, New York

Sherry Smith, RN, MSN, MBA
Senior Vice President of Clinical Operations
Intellicare, Inc
Portland, Maine

Christine Terenzi, RN, BSN, CEN
Clinical Educator
Emergency Department

Tacoma General Hospital
Tacoma, Washington

David Thompson, MD
Assistant Medical Director
Department of Emergency Medicine
MacNeal Hospital
Berwyn, Illinois

Eileen VanNorman, RN, CIC
Infection Control & Employee Health Nurse
ViaHealth of Wayne
Newark, New York

REVIEWERS *of the First Edition*

Samuel S. Bean, RN, MS
Wayne Regional Orthopaedic Associates
Immediate Past Director of Emergency Nursing
Myers Community Hospital
Sodus, New York

Julie Briggs, RN, BSN, MHA
Director of Emergency and Critical Care
  Services
Good Samaritan Hospital
Puyallup, Washington

Frank J. Edwards, MD, FACEP
Clinical Assistant Professor of Emergency
  Medicine
University of Rochester School of Medicine
Director, Division of Community and Rural
  Emergency Medicine of ViaHealth
Rochester, New York

Kevin Hanna, MD
Community and Rural Emergency Medicine of
  ViaHealth
Myers Community Hospital
Sodus, New York

R. Thomas Huntley
Public Health Regional Supervisor
Sexually Transmitted Disease Control Program
New York State Health Department
Syracuse, New York

Merrill Beth Kotok, RN C
Fetal Monitoring Unit
University of Rochester
Strong Memorial Hospital
Rochester, New York

Neal L. McGregor, PhD(c)
Professor of Religion and Business
Graceland College
Lamoni, Iowa

Margaret M. McMahon, RN, MN, CEN
Clinical Educator
Emergency Services
Atlantic City Medical Center
Atlantic City, New Jersey

Susan Spinello, CRNP, MSN, CEN, CCRN
Clinical Specialist
Emergency Department
University of Pennsylvania Medical Center
Philadelphia, Pennsylvania

Joseph Stamm, OD, FAAO
Private Practice
Clinical Associate, Department of
 Ophthalmology
University of Rochester School of Medicine
Rochester, New York

Marcia Ullman, RN, MS
Associate Professor of Psychiatric Nursing
State University of New York
College at Brockport
Brockport, New York

ILLUSTRATOR

John F. Aarne
Macedon, New York

PREFACE

Keeping pace with the ever-changing health care arena is a challenge for experienced health care professionals. The venture of entering a new environment in health care can seem overwhelming.

A common thread for anyone entering a patient care setting as the new team member is the need for user-friendly information. Facilities are well supplied with policy and procedure books and reference material for caregivers to refer to when clinical or administrative questions arise. New orientees and seasoned colleagues are often encouraged to create and carry "note cards" in their pockets or utilize a hand held computer notebook. These tools are highly individualized to the learning and practicing needs of each person.

Quick Reference to Triage (2nd edition), in essence, takes those note cards and compiles them into one source. It features a user-friendly format, allowing the busy health care professional to quickly glance at a page and determine immediately what should be assessed and considered for each patient. Over time, some of this material will be committed to memory . . . and some won't.

New additions to this book include information on maintaining safety while caring for members of gangs in your department, the evolving world of body mutilation (art, piercings, and implants), the new awareness our communities must have with regards to terrorist acts, as well as many other topics which have been asked for by our readers.

For consistency, the wording of the text refers to the emergency department setting. The material in this book is entirely appropriate for urgent care centers, private offices, schools, home health care agencies, prisons, and any other outpatient setting where patient assessment and triage occur.

ACKNOWLEDGMENTS

The completion of this book is due to the commitment and dedication of many wonderful people.

I am most grateful to my panel of reviewers and to my editor (Alan Sorkowitz) at Lippincott Williams & Wilkins. These groups of dedicated professionals maintained high standards and expectations for this text, were meticulously attentive to detail and deadlines, and believed in the investment this book required of all of us.

My sincere appreciation to Barb and Paul Bauer, Mimi Bennett, Laura Bouwens, Helen Breton, Julie Briggs, Betty Burns, Barb Grossklags, Donna Ojanen-Thomas, Gail Pisarcik-Lenehan, Neal McGregor, Sherry Smith, Carol Stock, David Thompson, and Linda Yee who have been encouraging and supportive mentors and friends to me through so many of the professional projects I find myself involved in.

A warm-hearted note of recognition to Shelley Cohen and Rebecca McNair, who share the passion of triage with me, and who have dedicated their careers to the education of nurses in the triage role.

Lastly, a special thanks to some of the best nurses I've ever rubbed elbows with, for teaching me every day how to improve my care of patients and for sharing the joy of our profession together . . . Doris Buschbascher, Kathy Fowler, Judy Gierstner, Greta Logue, Tracy Merrell, Stan Ryther, Judy Stone, Cindy Witter, and Tom Yale.

CONTENTS

Triage Process

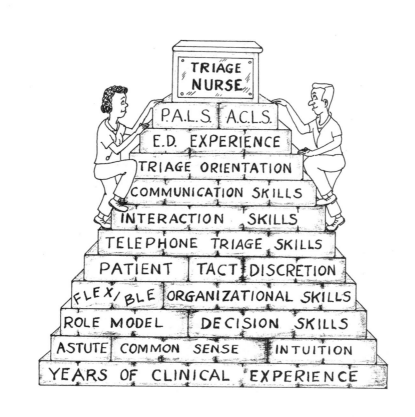

Notes

▶ FROM BATTLEFIELD TO FACILITY

Triage is derived from the French word, "trier," meaning to sort out. It was first used by the French military during World War I, when victims were sorted and classified according to the type and urgency of their conditions for the purpose of determining medical treatment priorities. The military intent was to provide care to the most treatable casualties so that soldiers could quickly return to the war front. Combat triage was guided by the adage "the best for the most with the least by the fewest." Critical patients requiring extensive resources received delayed medical care.

Lessons learned from wartime triaging are useful in the public sector. Triage is now used to organize the medical care available during disasters and mass casualty situations, and in emergency departments, urgent care centers, physicians' offices, and over the telephone.

Emergency Department (ED) use of triage systems began in the early 1960s, when the demand for emergency services outpaced available emergency resources. Emergency department space, equipment, and personnel were not adequate to handle the explosive increase in the number of emergency department visits. The rise in the number of ED visits was the result of many factors, including:

▲ more patients seeking treatment for nonurgent conditions
▲ patients with no other access to health care
▲ an increasing population sustaining a higher acuity of acute and chronic illnesses
▲ the negative impact from the rising use of illicit drugs
▲ an increase in the incidence of violent crime and trauma

As the use of EDs increased and the waiting times became longer, the triage process evolved as a way to effectively separate those patients requiring immediate medical attention from those who could wait. Triage in health care facilities differs in both purpose and function from that on the battlefield or at the disaster site. Emergency Department triage has become a major component of the emergency medical system and an expected standard of emergency nursing practice.

The primary goals of an effective ED triage system are to:

▲ *quickly* identify those patients with emergent, life-threatening conditions
▲ regulate the flow of patients through the ED
▲ provide direction to visitors and other health care professionals

An efficient triage system increases the quality of patient care delivered, shortens the length of a patient's stay, and decreases patient waiting time by combining immediate assessment and interventions. Organized triage categories are used to rate patient acuity, and standards are followed for assessment, planning, and intervention. Protocols are used for the initiation of specific diagnostic tests, medication administration, and treatments.

The advantages of triage include:

▲ The patient is greeted by a registered professional nurse, who establishes immediate communication, rapport, and sensitivity to the patient's and family's needs. The image of the facility is enhanced through positive client perceptions.
▲ Patient stress and anxiety are reduced when there is immediate contact with the nurse. The patient gains comfort knowing he or she is "in the system."
▲ Initial patient communication with the hospital, via the triage nurse, does not concern insurance or the ability to pay. This instills confidence in the patient that the ED is genuinely concerned with health problems and less concerned with ability to pay for the service received.

▲ Treatment of the patient requiring immediate care is expedited by the use of an acuity category system.

▲ Immediate assessment and documentation of patient problems are provided, while certain diagnostic procedures and treatments can be initiated without delay.

▲ Continuous reassessment of the ED patient who is waiting to be seen and continued communication with waiting family and friends ensure the delivery of quality care.

QUALITIES OF THE TRIAGE NURSE

The triage nurse is the first health care professional seen by the patient in the ED. Hospital surveys have shown that patient satisfaction with the ED and the hospital as a whole can be influenced by the initial encounter with the triage nurse.

The triage nurse must be sensitive to the patient's perception of the *health crisis* **that brought him or her to the ED.** The triage nurse must help the patient regain control and increase the understanding of his or her own health care role. Triage begins the process of managing a person's crisis instead of merely reacting to the situation.

Essential to the building of rapport between the triage nurse and the patient is the patient's first impression. The triage nurse has one opportunity to make a first impression on the patient. While in the waiting room or approaching the registration desk, the patient has the opportunity to view the triage nurse "on stage." The patient begins to develop an impression of the nurse before the first interaction even occurs. For this reason, it is vital for the triage nurse to act in a professional manner 100% of the time. The patient needs to know that the nurse is a genuinely concerned expert ready to assist in the patient's health care.

When greeting an incoming patient, the triage nurse must introduce her- or himself to the patient. Most patients will be unaware of what a triage nurse is or what the ED care process will be. This is an excellent opportunity for the triage nurse to "open the hospitality door" for the patient, begin the triage assessment, and educate the patient as to what can be expected during the ED visit.

The triage nurse acts as a positive influence for the patient by offering comfort and by communicating with the person in crisis. A guiding hand, a gentle voice tone, a warm smile, and attention to basic comfort needs (e.g., offering to carry coats or a parent's diaper bag) create an environment of true caring for the patient and family members.

Multi-situational organization and communication skills are essential for the triage nurse. Although the nurse may have to handle many different chaotic events at once, he or she must always make the patient in the triage room feel important. The triage nurse must be skilled in quality customer service, able to balance it all with graceful expertise—ringing telephones, ambulances, police, hospital colleagues, news media, and those in the waiting room.

The triage nurse encounters many people in the course of a shift. An unbiased and open mind is essential. The nurse must practice in an accepting manner, regardless of the cultural, religious, or social differences of the patients seeking care in the ED.

Much of the background for triage nursing is drawn from common sense. The basis for this comes from years of clinical experience, a broad range of nursing and medical knowledge, and extensive experience in dealing with emergency patients. These experiences, coupled with a working knowledge of ED routines, policies, and procedures, lead to a competent and efficient triage nurse.

The general qualifications strongly recommended for all nurses performing in the triage role, include:

▲ 6 to 12 months of emergency nursing experience
▲ demonstrated mastery of the hospital ED's competency-based orientation program
▲ Advanced Cardiac Life Support certification
▲ Pediatric Advanced Life Support certification
▲ certification in Emergency Nursing
▲ Emergency Nurses Pediatric Course completion
▲ precision assessment skills
▲ Trauma Nurse core curriculum
▲ working knowledge of intradepartmental policies
▲ ability to supervise others and delegate appropriately
▲ understanding of local emergency services (ambulance, police, helicopter, etc.)
▲ excellent telephone communication skills

Personal qualifications include:

▲ expertise in utilizing interpersonal and communication skills
▲ expertise in working collaboratively with others
▲ flexibility and adaptability, to meet the challenge of rapidly changing situations
▲ ability to act as a role model
▲ ability to utilize decision-making skills
▲ ability to anticipate future events and plan for potential occurrences
▲ mature understanding of conflict resolution
▲ well-developed skills in handling patients with special needs or barriers such as:
  • non-English speaking
  • expressive aphasia
  • intoxication from alcohol or other drugs
  • belligerent, hostile, or aggressive behavior
  • hearing or sight impairment
  • mental handicap
  • hysterical, crying, or panicky emotional state

To be a good triage nurse is to be a skilled, astute, compassionate health care professional with a great deal of common sense and intuition. It is one of the ultimate challenges in emergency nursing.

► CUSTOMER SERVICE

The professional health care staff must take a proactive role in offering high-quality customer service to patients, families, visitors, and colleagues. The excitement and challenge of the ED setting that attract the attention of many health care professionals also create difficulty in many of the interactions with those around us.

Chaos, crisis, noise, crowds, and high acuity are commonplace for ED professionals. For those other people who "visit" our department, those situations are sources of stress that add to the already difficult or unpleasant situation that brought them to the ED for service in the first place.

The triage nurse can create a positive environment by realizing that what may be normal for ED professionals is actually a great stressor for visitors. Whether it is a consulting physician in the department to see a patient or a family member worried about a loved one, it is the responsibility of the ED team member to welcome them into the department and express a sincere desire to facilitate their care and understanding.

▲ Start off your relationship with people in a warm, friendly manner.
  • Unhappy or stressed people can often be cheered up or comforted by a simple smile.
  • The patient carries more baggage than just a toothbrush packed in an overnight bag.
  • Help your visitor to deal with difficulties, just as you would comfort your own grandmother during a difficult time in her life.
▲ Be personal with people to help to create a sense of warmth.
  • Address your client by name and title (i.e., Mr. Jones) unless otherwise directed by the patient to use the first name.
  • Always be sure to introduce yourself by name and title.
  • Your clients will feel comforted just knowing an ED team member by name and feel protected that somebody seems to be watching over them.
▲ Offer assistance at every opportunity.
  • By expressing a sincere desire to help, the ED nurse builds a bridge to the patient and his or her family.
  • Once they understand that you are actively trying to help them, patients will often cooperate more readily with whatever requests you make, and reward you with their gratitude.
▲ *Simple manners* on the part of the ED staff, such as saying "*please*" and "*thank you*," outwardly illustrate your respect.
▲ Be honest and communicate frequently.
  • Your patient and his or her family seek the same goals health professionals do and deserve to be a part of the process.
  • Their stress level is already peaking, and lack of communication intensifies their situation.
▲ Always be proactive.
  • When a person appears upset, angry or sad, take a deep breath, walk over to him or her, put a smile on your face, and acknowledge his or her feelings.
  • The extra effort put forth and invested by the ED staff person initially often repays itself many times over in the long run.
  • In some cases, your efforts may go unrewarded, but at least you will have the satisfaction of knowing that you have tried your best.

No matter what your shift is like, there is always an opportunity to welcome those persons who are not members of your team and to teach them about who you are. You have the unique opportunity to provide everything from life-saving procedures to warm hospitality. Emergency Department professionals are members of a quality team, and this is an opportunity to show the world just how fine your team is.

▶ TRIAGE COURSE

The triage evaluation is an assessment process that collects objective and subjective information. The interview and physical assessment at triage must be reasonably comprehensive yet fit into a 4- or 5-minute time period. A complete head-to-toe assessment is usually neither feasible nor necessary.

The triage nurse practices within guidelines established by hospital, state, and federal agencies. To maintain compliance with established laws and regulations, the ED nurse performing triage is held to a degree of excellence that must always be maintained.

All patients presenting for care should be triaged on arrival (usually within 5 minutes) and receive a triage evaluation by the nurse before speaking with registration personnel. Patients presenting to the ED are always entitled to receive care in the ED, regardless of their ability to pay for service.

During times of extremely high patient volume, when the existing triage system is overloaded and patients are waiting an excessive amount of time to be evaluated by the nurse, the triage nurse on duty is responsible for getting assistance in the triage area. Each facility should have an overflow procedure in place that may include:

▲ having the ED technician obtain vital signs for each patient in triage while the nurse continues patient assessments
▲ requesting assistance from another ED nurse on duty
▲ requesting assistance from the ED charge nurse or other supervisory person

The triage assessment is the first segment of care the patient receives. It provides enough data to determine patient acuity and any immediate physiologic, psychological, psychosocial, or educational needs. Additionally, the information gathered by the triage nurse can be used for starting treatment or diagnostic testing from the triage office, following established protocols that the facility may have in place. These may include x-rays, administration of antipyretics, or diphtheria-tetanus immunization.

The triage nurse is responsible for assigning patients to an appropriate treatment area. In cases in which there is a question as to the level of triage acuity, the choice should be made favoring the more urgent assignment of care.

The triage nurse or the ED nurse taking over the care of that patient should ensure that reassessment occurs for each patient waiting to be seen by the physician. The assigned acuity level must be updated continually to include a change in the patient status or new information provided by the patient or family.

HOSPITAL RECEPTIONIST

There are times when the first employee a client may meet is the receptionist at the front desk, usually situated at or close to the front entrance. This person is generally responsible for greeting the incoming patient or visitor in a friendly manner, welcoming the patient to the facility, and assisting him or her with directions.

When the person presenting to this desk is sick or injured and seeking directions to the ED, the hospital receptionist must carefully guide the way. There are times, however, when the patient should not continue toward the ED without the assistance of a trained medical person in attendance.

The hospital receptionist is generally untrained in the recognition of medical emergencies. Training and on-the-job experience increase the receptionist's ability to determine those patients who "look sicker" than most.

Table 1–1 is designed to assist the hospital receptionist in determining how the patient should be guided to the ED, or if a medically trained person should be contacted immediately. It is based on the complaint (usually in one or two words) that the patient describes to the receptionist on arrival.

TABLE 1-1 • Guidelines for the Recognition of Medical Emergencies

Call for Emergency Response "Code Blue"	Call RN Immediately	Send Patient to Triage Area; Notify RN
Lifeless child carried in	Chest pain	Nausea, vomiting, diarrhea
Lifeless adult carried in	Difficulty breathing	"Cold" symptoms
	Gunshot wound	Minor wound, cut, bite
	Stab wound	Sore throat
	Seizure	Earache
	Massive bleeding	Bruise
	Difficulty staying awake	Minor sprain, strain
	Severe allergic reaction	
	Attempted suicide	
	Active labor	
	Active childbirth	
	Exposed broken bone	
	Violent patient	
	Eye injury (vision loss)	
	Large burn	
	Fever over 104°F	
	MVA/multiple trauma victim	

POINTS TO REMEMBER:
• Call the RN if there are any questions.
• Help the patient who needs assistance (wheelchair, etc.).
• Receptionist must not triage the patient or render medical advice.

INTERVIEW

The triage nurse should always begin the triage interview by introducing him- or herself by name and title. This provides the patient with the following:

▲ confidence that he or she is receiving care from a registered professional nurse
▲ the opportunity of open communication with the RN
▲ an additional degree of comfort, knowing that he or she can now identify with a member of the team by name

The triage interview is the basis for gathering data and making clinical decisions regarding the patient's acuity and need for intervention. The nurse elicits:

▲ chief complaints
▲ subjective and objective information pertinent to the presenting problem by utilizing the sense of:
  • sight
  • smell
  • hearing
  • intuition
  • touch

LOOK at the patient.

▲ Keen observation reveals:
- fear
- anxiety
- deformities
- respiratory problems
- obvious bleeding
- abnormal gait
- poor personal hygiene
- changes in skin color
- innumerable other signs

SMELL the patient's odors.

▲ The seasoned triage nurse is able to identify:
- alcohol
- marijuana
- ketone bodies
- incontinence
- ingested substances or poisons
- purulent infectious process

▲ The nurse must be sensitive to a host of smells that indicate different directions of treatment modalities.

LISTEN to what the patient and family are saying and to what they *are not* saying.

▲ The triage nurse uses the sense of hearing to assess:
- pain
- fear
- gross rales
- coughing
- shortness of breath
- a muffled voice
- family dynamics
- other indicators of a problem

TOUCH is instrumental in many ways.

▲ The sense of touch can assess:
- temperature
- sensation
- moisture
- "where it hurts"
- capillary refill
- soft tissue swelling

▲ By taking a radial pulse, the nurse can assess heart rate, possible cardiac arrhythmia, skin temperature, turgor, etc.

▲ Touch can also be:
  • psychologically therapeutic
  • used as an evaluation tool
  • used to communicate

Intuition plays a strong role in decisions made during triage.

  ▲ Intuition is a "sixth sense" that a patient:
  • is experiencing a problem that is more serious than it appears
  • is at risk for certain complications
  • needs particular attention to a set of symptoms
  ▲ This *unexplained sense* that results in the nurse assigning the patient to the ED as a more acute patient is based on:
  • in-depth knowledge of diseases and injuries
  • educational opportunities encountered throughout one's career
  • years of experience
  • CQI (continuous quality improvement) of presentations during triage evaluation of patients
  • a wide range of patients, disease processes, injuries, and variable presentation seen over a period of many years

To gather pertinent information, the triage interview should always be conducted with open-ended questions and with an open mind.

▶ PHYSICAL ASSESSMENT

Physical assessment accompanies the triage interview and often occurs while the nurse is obtaining the history. The physical assessment should be rapid, concise, and focused. The nurse performing triage should always begin with the primary survey (airway, breathing, and circulation), followed by the secondary survey. Box 1–1 depicts the PQRSTT mnemonic, which is helpful in systematically evaluating the presenting system.

By using the eyes, ears, nose, hands, and intuition, the triage nurse is able to have an accurate idea whether this patient requires immediate care or can wait the turn in line. Remember, make a triage decision, not a diagnosis.

▶ BASIC TRIAGE ASSESSMENT

All patients presenting to the ED have a routine triage assessment performed, including a primary and a focused secondary assessment. All findings must be accurately documented. Depending on facility policy, obtain the following information:

  ▲ Patient name (ask patient for correct spelling)
  ▲ Date and time of initial patient contact with triage nurse
  ▲ Mode of arrival (walk, wheelchair, car, or ambulance)
  ▲ Age in years (if >2 years old) or in months (if <24 months)
  ▲ Chief complaint of the patient, usually two to three quoted words from patient

■ Box 1–1: **THE PQRSTT MNEMONIC**

P = Provoking factors

- What makes it (pain, breathing, etc.) worse?
- What makes it better?
- Any known trauma or injury?

Q = Quality of pain

- What does it feel like?
- Does the patient use descriptive words such as burning, stabbing, crushing, or tearing?

R = Region/Radiation

- Where is the pain?
- Is it in one spot?
- Does it start in one spot and travel to another?
- Ask the patient to point to where it hurts using one finger.

S = Severity of pain

- If the patient were to describe the pain with a number from 1 to 10, with 1 being the least severe and 10 being the worst pain imaginable, what number would the patient give this pain?

T = Time

- When did this start?
- How long have the symptoms persisted?
- How long did it last?
- Has it ever happened before?

T = Treatment

- Has the patient taken any medication to treat this?
- What time was the last dose?
- Has the patient done anything to treat him- or herself?
- What has or has not worked for the patient?

▲ Applicable past history including:
  - medical
  - surgical
  - orthopedic
  - psychiatric
  - obstetric/gynecologic/GU
    - sexual activity
    - form of birth control
    - chance of current pregnancy
    - last use of Viagra (in men presenting with chest pain)
▲ Brief triage history and physical assessment per protocol
  - What happened?
  - When did it happen?
  - Where does it hurt?

▲ Current medication taken by patient, including:
  - over-the-counter medication
  - prescription medication
  - tobacco use
  - alcohol use
  - illicit drug use
  - herbal or alternative healing methods
  - Viagra within past 24 hours (ACC/AHA, 1999)
  - risk of "date rape" drug ingestion
▲ Allergies to medication, including the reaction (rash, respiratory distress, etc.)
  - some facilities use red ink for documenting allergies
  - assess for latex allergy on all patients by asking, "Have you ever developed itching, burning, swelling, or hives after blowing up a balloon or wearing rubber gloves?"
▲ Immunization status for all patients less than 18 years old per protocol and last dT for all patients more than 18 years old regardless of complaint. (Refer to the immunization schedule in the pediatric Pearls of Triage Wisdom, later in the book.)
▲ First day of the last normal menstrual period (LNMP) for all women of childbearing age
▲ Weight for all pediatric patients
  - consider risk of eating disorders for all ages
▲ Vital signs, per departmental policy
▲ Triage acuity assessment and documentation per protocol
▲ Glasgow Coma Scale (GCS) and/or Trauma Score (TS) for all trauma patients, altered LOC, head injury patients, etc.
▲ Signature of triage nurse (including first initial, last name, and credentials)

Orthostatic Vital Signs

Orthostatic vital signs can be a beneficial assessment tool for the triage nurse in assigning acuity levels to triaged patients. Orthostatic vital signs should be assessed on all patients who present with:

▲ vomiting
▲ fever
▲ diarrhea
▲ abdominal pain
▲ dizziness
▲ syncope
▲ weakness
▲ bleeding (especially vaginal)

 ALERT **Caution:** If a patient looks hemodynamically unstable, has a possible or probable spinal injury, or has an altered level of consciousness, the triage nurse should defer obtaining orthostatic vital signs until *after* the patient is evaluated by the physician.

To perform this procedure:
1. The patient should rest in the supine position for 3 to 5 minutes.
2. After this rest, obtain blood pressure (BP) and pulse with the patient supine.
3. Slowly assist the patient to a sitting position, with feet dangling over the bedside.
4. Allow the patient to remain in this sitting position for 1 minute.
5. After this rest, obtain BP and pulse with the patient in the sitting position.
6. Slowly assist the patient to a standing position.
7. Allow the patient to remain standing for 1 minute.
8. After this rest, obtain BP and pulse.
9. Assess how the patient tolerated the procedure (asymptomatic, became dizzy, etc.).

To document this procedure:
1. Indicate the time of the procedure.
2. Indicate if the patient experienced symptoms during the procedure.
3. Document each BP and pulse for each position.

Example:

8:30 AM	lying:	140/68;	HR 82
	sitting:	136/66;	HR 90
	standing:	128/62;	HR 100

Stick figures, instead of the written word, may be used for documentation purposes when describing the different positions.

A "positive" result would show:

▲ a rise in the pulse of >20 beats per minute
▲ a fall in the systolic blood pressure of >20 mmHg
▲ a fall in the diastolic blood pressure of >10 mmHg

Orthostatic vital signs can be partially utilized in the triage room, especially during times of high volume and acuity in the department. By performing the sitting and standing portion of this procedure, the triage nurse is able to assess the patient's acuity level more precisely and make a more accurate decision regarding the priority of care (Blazys, 2000).

Orthostatic vital signs are also utilized during the ongoing care of patients. The nurse may decide to utilize them as a part of the ongoing assessment process of the patient in addition to their use during triage or when specifically requested by the physician.

Orthostatic vital signs should be considered as part of the reassessment of:

▲ patients receiving IV hydration
▲ patients who had "positive" orthostatic vital signs on arrival
▲ patients who received medication that could cause drowsiness or other central nervous system (CNS) depression

Pain Assessment

The primary reason most patients come to the ED seeking care is because "something hurts." For years, emergency care has focused primary importance on treating those patients in need of "resuscitative or emergent" care.

Pain, however, is a very important part of patient care. It is essential for the emergency staff to focus on the patient's perception of his or her pain and help to address that pain.

ACUTE AND CHRONIC PAIN

Acute pain:

- ▲ is often a warning sign that something is wrong
- ▲ may last for hours, days, or weeks before the patient seeks care and is associated with:
  - tissue injury
  - inflammation
  - surgical procedures
  - disease process

Chronic pain is:

- ▲ long-lasting, and may worsen or intensify over months, years, or a lifetime, and is associated with:
  - cancer
  - HIV/AIDS
  - arthritis
  - fibromyalgia
  - diabetes
  - injury (e.g., low-back pain)
  - reflex sympathetic dystrophy
  - phantom limb pain

WILDA

Pain should be assessed on a regular basis and be individualized to the patient. A standard approach should be used, so that each caretaker of the patient will be able to perform a pain assessment in a similar manner, and trending will occur as a result.

One method of pain assessment is the WILDA approach to pain assessment. The mnemonic stands for:

W	=	**W**ords
I	=	**I**ntensity
L	=	**L**ocation
D	=	**D**uration
A	=	**A**ggravating/Alleviating Factors

Words

Patients may not be able to fully describe their pain on their own. The health care professional should assist them with the description through appropriate interviewing techniques. Ask open-ended questions and do not hesitate to ask the patient to find more than one word to describe the pain.

Possible words used to describe pain include:

- ▲ aching
- ▲ burning
- ▲ cramping

▲ deep
▲ dull
▲ gnawing
▲ numb
▲ pressure
▲ radiating
▲ shooting
▲ smarting
▲ sore
▲ squeezing
▲ stabbing
▲ stinging
▲ tender
▲ throbbing
▲ tingling
▲ twinge

Health care professionals may better assist their patients if a basic understanding of pain types is available.

▲ Neuropathic pain
  • Caused by nerve disorders or injuries
  • Described as:
    – burning
    – shooting
    – tingling
    – radiating
▲ Somatic pain
  • Localized pain that accompanies orthopedic concerns such as arthritis, bone metastases, low-back pain, or orthopedic injuries or procedures
  • Described as:
    – aching
    – throbbing
    – dull
▲ Visceral pain
  • Occurs with thoracic or abdominal issues
  • Described as:
    – squeezing
    – pressure
    – cramping
    – dull
    – deep

Intensity

A universal scale of pain quantification is the standard "rate your pain on a scale from 0 to 10." This by itself does not provide the information that the health care team needs to fully evaluate the patient's pain. Be sure to additionally ascertain the following information from the patient by asking "How would you rate your . . ."

- ▲ present pain?
- ▲ pain after interventions?
- ▲ during the past 24 hours?

In addition to determining the level of pain the patient is experiencing, inquire whether this level of pain is acceptable to him or her. Be sure to discuss mutual goals in pain relief with the patient (e.g., Total pain relief? Enough relief to walk?)

Location

Ask for specific details when determining the location of patients' pain. Determine if they have pain in more than one spot, and have them describe the different types and locations of pain they are experiencing. Asking patients to "point to where it hurts with one finger" will assist the nurse in proper assessment, treatment, and documentation of patients' perceived pain.

Duration

Once pain treatment has been initiated, the nurse must reassess the patient's perception of pain. The pain may be constant, intermittent, or be different, depending on the location of the pain and the patient's activity at the time.

Aggravating/Alleviating Factors

Determine what makes the patient's pain worsen or improve. Discover how this pain influences life activities such as eating, working, sleeping, etc. Also determine if other symptoms occur when the pain is present (e.g., nausea, weakness, etc.)

Triage Documentation

The triage process is complete when the information elicited during the assessment process has been fully and accurately documented. Documentation on the patient's ED chart is crucial to support the decisions and actions of the triage nurse and the ED staff.

All pertinent information gathered during the triage process (interview history and physical assessment) must be documented. Pertinent negatives may also be listed, such as "denies nausea, vomiting, or fever." These are important pieces of necessary information when focusing on the patient's condition.

If nursing interventions took place during triage, documentation should reflect those. It is essential that every nursing intervention, from the administration of antipyretics to the seclusion of a patient in a quiet room, be appropriately recorded on the patient's medical record.

Assigning Acuity

- ▲ Triage acuity categories represent:
  - the acuity of each patient's condition
  - the anticipated amount of nursing care the patient will need while in the ED
  - a continuum in which one patient presents more emergent than another

▲ In cases where there is a question as to the level of triage acuity, the choice should be made toward the ***more serious*** category of care.
- Each ED should have its own patient classification system in place, which can be located in the ED policy book.
- The Emergency Nurses Association is moving towards a standard of a 5-tier acuity system.
  - A 5-tier system will allow greater accuracy when assigning an acuity to each patient and provide for greater reproducibility among a department's nursing staff.
  - It will also promote clearer communication between facilities and remove the guesswork that occurs when trying to compare a patient in a 3-tier system to a patient in a 5-tier system.
- Determining the acuity category for those patients in the middle of the continuum is a challenge for the triage nurse.

▲ The triage nurse should carefully consider those age-fragile patients (<12 months or >60 years old) who may be less able to tolerate the simpler injuries and illnesses, and may adjust the patient's acuity level to a more serious category.

▲ If a patient presents with more than one chief complaint or has comorbidities, the triage nurse must individually address each of the patient's concerns.
- The nurse may opt to place this patient in a higher acuity category, since the client's ED medical evaluation will probably be more detailed.

▲ The triage nurse applies subjective and objective data gathered to determine triage categories. For instance:
- On the basis of practical knowledge gained through experience and training, certain signs and symptoms trigger the triage nurse's suspicion toward a particular clinical impression.
  - Example: The 64-year-old male with chest pain and shortness of breath is classified as emergent because the nurse knows the probability of myocardial infarction in this patient and its potential complications.
- Discovery of a sign or symptom that will result in a poor outcome unless immediate care is rendered warrants a particular acuity category.
  - Example: Profuse bleeding or the presence of stridor directs the nurse to triage the patient as emergent.
- A standardized approach that promotes consistency and reliability throughout the ED nursing staff is attained by the triage nurse following established guidelines and triage protocols to determine the accurate triage acuity category. These guidelines promote early initiation of simple diagnostics, treatments, and patient teaching.

▲ It cannot be stressed enough that acuity categories are only a guideline.
- If the triage nurse believes that a patient needs to be placed at a higher level of acuity, it is within the realm of responsibilities of the triage nurse to do so.

▲ The triage nurse also must be careful of those patients who repeatedly visit the ED with minor complaints.
- Most psychoneurotic patients ultimately die from organic disease.
- We all remember the story about the boy who cried wolf. We are now in a position to adapt to and care for these patients who may not always be the easiest or most pleasant individuals.

▲ Patients who return to the ED within 72 hours are known to be high-risk patients.
- These patients may have a more progressive or severe medical condition than originally identified during their first visit.
- They may be dissatisfied with previous care received or are seeking a second opinion.

- These patients must receive a complete medical screening exam by the ED physician *each* and *every* time they present to the ED.
▲ There are a variety of different triage models to follow, using three, four, or five acuity categories (Tables 1–2, 1–3, and 1–4).

TABLE 1–2 • Five-Level Acuity System

Level	Acuity	Treatment and Reassessment Time	Sample Conditions	
Level 1	Resuscitative	Immediately	Cardiac arrest Seizure Anaphylaxis Multiple trauma Profound shock Severe respiratory distress	Chest pain Uncontrolled hemorrhage Severe head trauma Open chest/abdominal wound Poisoning with neurologic changes
Level 2	Emergent	5–15 minutes	Major fracture Severe headache Aggressive patient Major burn Stroke Acute asthma attack Active labor patient	Drug overdose (tricyclic) Suicidal/homicidal behavior Sexual assault survivor Eye injury with vision loss Pregnant (active bleeding) Testicular pain (boys)
Level 3	Urgent	15–45 minutes	Alcohol/drug intoxication Drug ingestion Urinary retention Renal calculi Laceration Closed fracture	Noncardiac chest pain Severe emotional distress Minor chest pain Eye injury (vision intact) Bleeding (patient stable) Abdominal pain
Level 4	Semi-urgent	1–2 hours	Cystitis STDs Sore throat Abscess Minor burn	Minor bites Vaginal discharge Constipation Strain and sprains Earache
Level 5	Routine	4 hours	Routine physical Bruise	Suture removal Prescription refill

TABLE 1–3 • Four-Level Acuity System

Level	Acuity	Treatment and Reassessment Time	Sample Conditions
Level 1	Resuscitative	Immediately	Cardiac arrest Seizure Anaphylaxis Multiple trauma Profound shock Severe respiratory distress Chest pain Uncontrolled hemorrhage Severe head trauma Open chest/abdominal wound Poisoning with neurologic changes
Level 2	Emergent	5–15 minutes	Major fracture Severe headache Aggressive patient Major burn Stroke Acute asthma attack Active labor patient Drug overdose (tricyclic) Suicidal/homicidal behavior Sexual assault survivor Eye injury with vision loss Pregnant (active bleeding) Testicular pain (boys)
Level 3	Urgent	15–45 minutes	Alcohol/drug intoxication Drug ingestion Urinary retention Renal calculi Laceration Closed fracture Abdominal pain Noncardiac chest pain Severe emotional distress Minor chest pain Eye injury (vision intact) Bleeding (stable vital signs)
Level 4	Nonurgent	1–2 hours	Cystitis Sexually transmitted disease Sore throat Abscess Minor burn Minor bites (human, insect, animal) Vaginal discharge Constipation Strain and sprains Earache

TABLE 1-4 • **Three-Level Acuity System**

Level	Acuity	Treatment and Reassessment Time	Sample Conditions
Level 1	Resuscitative	Immediately	Cardiac arrest Seizure Anaphylaxis Multiple trauma Profound shock Severe respiratory distress Chest pain Uncontrolled hemorrhage Severe head trauma Open chest/abdominal wound Poisoning with neurologic changes Active labor patient Drug overdose (tricyclic)
Level 2	Emergent	10–45 minutes	Major fracture Severe headache Aggressive patient Major burn Stroke Acute asthma attack Urinary retention Renal calculi Laceration (serious) Suicidal/homicidal behavior Sexual assault survivor Eye injury with vision loss Pregnant (active bleeding) Testicular pain (boys) Alcohol/drug intoxication Drug ingestion
Level 3	Urgent	30 minutes–2 hours	Closed fracture Abdominal pain Noncardiac chest pain Severe emotional distress Minor chest pain Eye injury (vision intact) Bleeding (stable vital signs)

Triage Guidelines

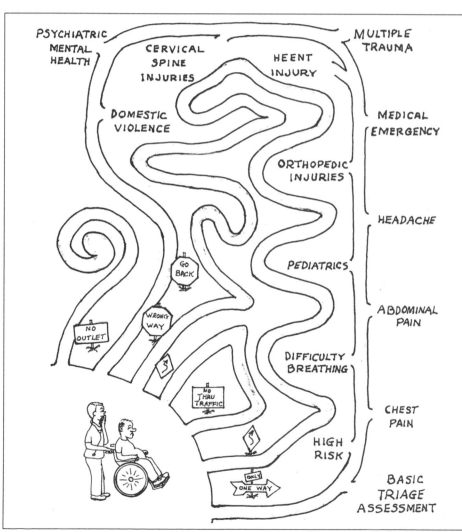

Notes

▶ ABDOMINAL PAIN (GI/GU)

Assessment

A. Obtain and record triage assessment that includes:
1. Description of pain:
   - ▲ **P**rovoking factors (what makes it better or worse?)
   - ▲ **Q**uality of pain
   - ▲ **R**egion/radiation
   - ▲ **S**everity of pain (1–10 scale)
   - ▲ **T**ime (onset, duration)
   - ▲ **T**reatment (what has the patient already tried?)
2. Associated symptoms (Table 2–1):
   - ▲ fever
   - ▲ nausea
   - ▲ vomiting
   - ▲ diarrhea
   - ▲ LNMP
   - ▲ chest pain
   - ▲ difficulty breathing
   - ▲ right shoulder pain
   - ▲ last bowel movement
   - ▲ urinary symptoms
   - ▲ penile discharge
   - ▲ scrotal pain or swelling
   - ▲ gravid history
   - ▲ sexual activity
   - ▲ vaginal discharge
3. Past medical/surgical history:
   - ▲ diabetes
   - ▲ similar history of abdominal pain
   - ▲ hypertension
   - ▲ abdominal surgeries
   - ▲ coronary artery disease
B. Complete basic triage assessment per protocol and **document** accurately.
C. Obtain orthostatic vital signs as indicated.
D. Consider obtaining clean-catch urine sample from female patients.
   - ▲ if suspicion of urinary tract infection, a portion of the sample may be dipstick tested, with results recorded on triage note
   - ▲ male patients presenting with possible STD symptoms **should not** obtain urine sample before physician exam

TABLE 2–1 • Differential Presentations of Abdominal Pain

Possible Diagnosis	Signs and Symptoms
Abdominal aortic aneurysm	• Asymptomatic until leakage or rupture occur • Abrupt onset of severe back, flank, or abdominal pain • Pulsatile abdominal mass, mottling of lower extremities, signs of shock
Appendicitis	• Diffuse pain in epigastric or periumbilical area for 1–2 days • Localization of pain over the right lower quadrant between the umbilicus and right iliac crest • Anorexia, nausea/vomiting, fever, tachycardia, pallor, peritoneal signs • Increased pain with stairs, walking, etc.
Bowel obstruction	• Severe, crampy, colicky abdominal pain • Vomiting, constipation, hypotension, tachycardia, abdominal distention, hyperactive bowel sounds, fever
Cholecystitis (inflammation of gallbladder)	• Colicky discomfort in the right upper-quadrant midepigastric area • Pain radiation to the shoulders and back • Nausea/vomiting, fever, tachycardia, tachypnea, abdominal guarding, jaundice, malaise
Cholelithiasis (presence of gallbladder stones)	• Severe, steady or colicky pain in the upper abdominal quadrant, often right-sided • Pain usually begins 3–6 hours after a large meal • Pain radiation to scapula, back, or right shoulder • Nausea, vomiting, dyspepsia, mild to moderate jaundice
Constipation/ fecal impaction	• Clinically defined as defecation less than three times per week • Each patient may interpret the symptoms differently • Fatigue, abdominal discomfort, headache, low back pain, anorexia, restlessness
Duodenal or ileojejunal hematoma	• Caused by a blow to the abdomen • Immediate bruising over upper quadrant of abdomen
Epididymitis	• Infection or inflammation of the epididymis • Swelling, enlargement of the epididymis, sudden swelling of the spermatic cord, fever, dysuria, urethral discharge
Intussusception	• Paroxysms of acute abdominal pain, intermittent with episodes of being pain free • Currant jelly, mucus-type stools or rectal bleeding • Fever, lethargy, vomiting (food, mucus, fecal matter), dehydration
Orchitis	• Inflammation or infection of the testicle • Intense pain and swelling of the scrotum, dysuria, urethral discharge, fever, discomfort in the groin/lower abdomen, acutely ill
Pancreatitis	• Severe, constant upper-quadrant midepigastric pain that radiates to the midback • Pain worsens when lying flat on back, relieved when lying on side with knees drawn up • Nausea, vomiting, fever, pallor, hypotension, tachycardia, tachypnea, restlessness, malaise, fatty or foul-smelling stools, abdominal distention, pulmonary crackles
Peritonitis	• Severe pain that gradually increases in intensity and worsens with movement • Riding in car, climbing stairs, or jumping on one foot greatly worsens pain • Radiation of pain to shoulder, back, or chest • Nausea, vomiting, fever, abdominal distention, rigidity, and tenderness

TABLE 2–1 • Differential Presentations of Abdominal Pain (Continued)

Possible Diagnosis	Signs and Symptoms
Renal calculi	• Location of stone depicts associated pain: flank, lower abdominal quadrant, low back, groin, testicular, labial or urethral meatus • Pain radiation varies depending on stone location • Nausea, vomiting, pale, diaphoretic, marked restlessness, dehydration
Ruptured ovarian cyst	• Sudden severe, unilateral lower-quadrant abdominal pain associated with exercise or intercourse • Delayed or prolonged menstruation, vomiting, ascites, signs of peritonitis
Tubal pregnancy	• Intermittent diffuse abdominal pain • Radiation of pain to shoulder • Vaginal spotting/bleeding, syncope, dizziness, signs of peritonitis or shock
Urinary tract infection	• Lower-quadrant abdominal or pelvic pain • Urinary burning, frequency, urgency, hematuria, foul-smelling urine, fever, bladder spasms
Cystitis	• Dysuria, urinary frequency and urgency, fever, hematuria
Pyelonephritis	• Flank or back pain • Urinary frequency, dysuria, fever, malaise, nausea, vomiting, chills
Prostatitis	• Perineal aching, low-back pain • Urinary frequency, dysuria, fever, malaise, urethral discharge, prostatic swelling
Testicular torsion	• Sudden onset of severe, unilateral testicular pain and tenderness • Nausea, vomiting, fever, scrotal mass
Ulcer: gastric duodenal esophageal	• Colicky, burning, squeezing pain in the epigastric or midback area • Pain intensity is variable, often begins 1–3 hours after meals, worsens at night • Nausea, vomiting, hematemesis, abdominal guarding, decreased or absent bowel sounds

Immediate Care If

- ▲ Age older than 50 years and/or any of the following:
  - syncope (actual or near)
  - hypertension
  - arteriosclerotic heart disease
  - diabetes
  - aneurysm
  - pain radiating into back or legs
  - lightheadedness
  - weakness/paresthesia of legs
  - systolic BP <100 or >160
  - pulse >100 or <60
  - any suspicion of AAA
- ▲ Heavy vaginal bleeding
- ▲ Young male with testicular pain or swelling
- ▲ Blood in emesis or stool (or suspicion of blood)
- ▲ Severe abdominal pain
- ▲ Unstable vital signs
- ▲ Persistent vomiting or profuse diarrhea:
  - more than 18 hours in patients older than 6 years
  - more than 12 hours in children less than 6 years old
  - more than 8 hours since last void
- ▲ Referral by PMD with possible:
  - acute abdomen
  - intestinal obstruction

ANKLE INJURIES

 Assessment

A. Obtain and record triage assessment that includes:
1. What happened?
   - ▲ description of injury
   - ▲ mechanism of injury
     - inversion (foot bends inward, ankle falls outward)
     - eversion (foot bends outward, ankle bends inward)
2. When did the injury occur?
3. Can the patient put weight on the foot? Ambulate?
4. Where is the point of maximum tenderness?
5. How is the circulation? Check:
   - ▲ capillary refill
   - ▲ pedal pulses
   - ▲ warm versus cool
   - ▲ normal skin color versus pallor
B. Perform physical assessment of foot and ankle, by palpating:
   - ▲ lateral aspect of foot and ankle
   - ▲ medial aspect of foot and ankle
   - ▲ midfoot region
   - ▲ fifth metatarsal
C. Complete remainder of basic triage assessment and **document** completely.

Immediate Care If

- ▲ Marked deformity of the foot or ankle
- ▲ Unstable foot or ankle joint
- ▲ Absence of pulses or prolonged capillary refill
- ▲ Open fracture
- ▲ Compartment syndrome noted

Interventions

1. If triage assessment reveals a stable ankle, place patient in wheelchair, elevate affected leg, and apply ice to area.
   - ▲ Order x-ray of ankle (if your facility's protocol permits) if there is:
     - marked malleolar or submalleolar swelling/ecchymosis
     - history of severe pain when trying to bear weight
   - ▲ Order x-ray of foot (if your facility's protocol permits) if there is:
     - a crush-type injury with midfoot swelling
     - swelling over the base of the fifth metatarsal
   - ▲ Refrain from ordering x-ray if:
     - patient can reasonably bear weight
     - malleoli are not tender
     - no instability is noted
2. If triage assessment reveals an unstable ankle:
   - ▲ Place patient on a stretcher immediately.
   - ▲ Apply ice to the area.
   - ▲ Splint the joint with pillow or other available splint.
   - ▲ Notify ED physician.

BURN TRAUMA

Facts

On an annual basis:

- ▲ More than 2 million burn injuries occur.
- ▲ 1.25 million burn injuries require medical attention.
- ▲ 500,000 ED visits result from burn injuries.
- ▲ 25,000 patients are admitted to specialized burn units.
- ▲ More than 4,500 patients will die as a result of their burn injury (NIGMS, 2001).
- ▲ Different types of burn injury include:
  - inhalation
  - thermal
  - electrical
  - chemical
  - radiation
- ▲ Burns initiate an inflammatory response of the affected area of the body, resulting in heat, redness, swelling, and pain.
- ▲ When the skin is burned, the following functions are altered:
  - sensation
  - skin regeneration
  - body temperature
  - conservation and balances of body fluids
  - body image and self-esteem
  - protection against infection and injury

General Issues

 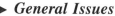

Assessment

A. Complete appropriate triage assessment protocol and **document** carefully.
  - ▲ basic triage assessment (important to determine underlying medical conditions)
  - ▲ multiple trauma (one third of burn patients have other injuries)
  - ▲ pediatric trauma
  - ▲ domestic violence and child abuse

B. Assess burn wound.
  - ▲ type
  - ▲ location
  - ▲ blisters

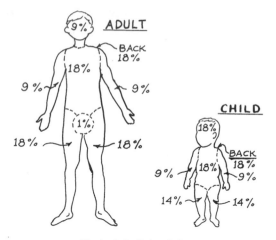

Figure 2–1. Rule of nines.

▲ appearance (e.g., blanching)
▲ extent (rule of nines—Figure 2–1)
▲ depth (first-, second-, or third-degree—Table 2–2)
C. Determine severity of burn injury and percentage of each type.

TABLE 2–2 • Burn Identification				
Depth	*Degree*	*Appearance*	*Associated Pain*	*Healing Process*
Partial thickness—epidermal	1st	Red and dry No blisters Blanches to pressure	Painful	3–5 days
Partial thickness—superficial	1st–2nd	Red to pale ivory color Weeping blisters Blanches to pressure	Increased sensitivity to: • pain • pressure • temperature	10 days–3 weeks

Partial thickness—deep	2nd–3rd	Mottled, white waxy
		  blisters
		Bullae
			Depending on
			  the depth, may
			  be **very** painful
			  or decreased
			  sensitivity to:
			• pain
			• pressure
			• temperature
				Several weeks
				to months

Full thickness	3rd	Dry, white Charred, leathery Does not blanch	Absent sensitivity to: • pain • pressure • temperature	Skin grafting required

Interventions

Vary depending on the severity and type of the burn injury

1. Establish and maintain ABCs.
2. Insert IV access using large-bore catheters (14–16 gauge) on unburned areas.
   ▲ Burned areas may be used if necessary, or may need cutdown by physician.
3. Replace fluid volume deficit with lactated Ringer's solution (adult and child).
   ▲ Usual replacement formula for first 24 hours post–burn injury is *4 cc LR X kg X % of burn (up to 50% max)*.
   ▲ Infuse as follows:
   - *first 8 hours* after burn: administer one half of calculated IV replacement
   - *second 8 hours* after burn: administer one quarter of calculated IV replacement
   - *third 8 hours* after burn: administer one quarter of calculated IV replacement
4. Monitor and maintain urine output:
   ▲ Adults: 30–50 ml/hr (0.5–1.0 ml/kg/hr)
   ▲ Children: <30 kg: 1.0 ml/kg/hr
5. Perform initial wound care:
   ▲ If wound is still warm, apply cool, moist, sterile compress for no longer than 15 minutes to minor burns (<10% in age fragile, <15% in adults).
   ▲ *Never* place ice on a burn wound.
   ▲ Offer pain management for all wound care procedures.
   ▲ Cleanse minor burn wounds with a nondetergent soap; the receiving burn team will usually cleanse major burns.
6. Consider use of documentation forms:
   ▲ Pediatric Injury Assessment
   ▲ Elder Abuse
   ▲ Rule of Nines
7. Consider and arrange for the transfer of patient to a burn center using the criteria shown in Table 2–3.

TABLE 2-3 • Criteria For Transfer to Burn Center

Age	Depth/Area of Body	% Total Body Surface Area (TBSA)
<10 years old	2nd and 3rd degree	>10
10–50 years old	2nd and 3rd degree	>20
>50 years old	2nd and 3rd degree	>10
any age	3rd degree	>5
any age	2nd or 3rd degree to the face, hands, feet, or genitalia	Any

- Consider transfer to a burn center for any of the following:
  - electrical burns (including lightning injury)
  - chemical burns
  - inhalation injury
  - comorbidities in a patient
    - pre-existing health issues
    - mental illness
    - multiple trauma

▶ *Inhalation Burn Injury*

Most deaths from fires occur from inhalation injuries.

Assessment

1. Assess the patient for:
   - ▲ laryngeal spasm
   - ▲ hoarseness
   - ▲ singed facial hair
   - ▲ facial burns
   - ▲ dysphagia
   - ▲ burning sensation in the throat or chest
   - ▲ dyspnea
   - ▲ cough
   - ▲ ashen skin
   - ▲ gray or black sputum
   - ▲ carbonaceous sputum
   - ▲ blisters in nose or mouth
   - ▲ singed nasal hair
   - ▲ uvula edema
   - ▲ hypoxia
   - ▲ pallor
   - ▲ cyanosis
   - ▲ soot around the nose or in the oropharynx

▶ *Carbon Monoxide Poisoning (Enclosed Exposure to Incomplete Combustion)*

Assessment

1. Determine what the patient was exposed to:
   - ▲ gas or propane
   - ▲ faulty furnace
   - ▲ fire
   - ▲ automobile exhaust
   - ▲ charcoal burner
   - ▲ stove
2. Obtain and evaluate carboxyhemoglobin saturation level, if needed (Table 2–4).

TABLE 2–4 • Carboxyhemoglobin Saturation Levels

Level (%)	Associated Indicators and Symptoms
0–5	Normal for nonsmokers
5–10	Normal for smokers
10–20	Headache, visual acuity impairment, irritability
20–30	Flushing, confusion
30–40	Nausea/vomiting, lack of coordination, dizziness, lethargy, ST segment depression
40–50	Chest pain, tachycardia, tachypnea, agitation
>50	Loss of consciousness, seizures, coma, death

Interventions

1. Provide 100% oxygen via mask until levels are below 10% to 20%.

Electrical Injury

The electrical current enters through the skin, converts to heat, passes through the body, and exits the body—thus producing entrance and exit burn wounds. Although the external burn wounds may appear minor, the notable injury occurs internally along the path created by the current, between the entrance and exit wounds.

- ▲ Low voltage (<600 volts)
  - • Household current is 110 to 220V and usually harmless
- ▲ High voltage (>600 volts)
  - • Most common in electrical and construction workers
  - • 3rd rail of a subway is 600 volts
  - • Residential power lines are 7620 volts
- ▲ Lightning
  - • Seen most often during summer months because of thunderstorm activity (Thompson, 2001)

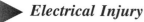

Assessment

1. Determine the following:
   - ▲ path of the current
   - ▲ duration of contact
   - ▲ intensity and type of current
     - • low voltage
     - • high voltage
     - • alternating current
     - • direct current
   - ▲ resistance of the tissues to the passage of current
2. Evaluate entrance/exit wounds

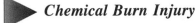

Interventions (In addition to previously discussed care)

1. Maintain ABCs.
2. Obtain cardiac enzymes.
3. Obtain 12-lead ECG.
4. Continue cardiac monitoring.

► *Chemical Burn Injury*

Assessment

1. Determine the following:
   - ▲ type of chemical
   - ▲ concentration
   - ▲ duration of contact
   - ▲ mechanism of injury
   - ▲ extent of tissue penetration

Interventions

1. Remove clothing from patient.
2. Lavage area with copious amount of water or saline:
   - ▲ 30 minutes for acid burns
   - ▲ 1 to 2 hours for alkaline burns

POSSIBLE CERVICAL SPINE INJURY (CONSIDER POSSIBILITY OF NECK INJURY WITH ANY OTHER INJURY)

Assessment

A. Obtain and record basic triage assessment that includes:
   1. Mechanism of injury
   2. Alteration in range of motion (do not test range of motion [ROM] of neck)
   3. Alteration in sensory perception
   4. Time of injury

Interventions

1. For patients presenting ambulatory to the ED, and there is an indication that a neck injury may have occurred, prepare for immediate immobilization of the patient's c-spine.
   ▲ Explain the importance of and the procedure for immobilization of the patient's c-spine.
   ▲ Obtain the correct size collar for the patient.
   ▲ Place collar on patient and secure appropriately.
   ▲ Immediately place the patient onto a stretcher (follow specific departmental policy for c-spine immobilization process in triage).
   ▲ Contact ED physician if not already involved in care of the patient.
   ▲ Clearly document the process of c-spine immobilization.
2. Complete remainder of basic triage assessment and document carefully.
3. Frequently observe and communicate with the patient.
   ▲ Place patient in room easily visible and audible from nurse's station.
   ▲ Educate patient (and visitors) of the importance of remaining supine on stretcher until c-spine is cleared by physician.
4. Keep patient NPO.
5. Have suction set up and ready for use at bedside.
6. Be prepared to log-roll patient:
   ▲ if patient vomits
   ▲ if physician needs assistance with examination of patient's back
7. Undress patient for physician evaluation:
   ▲ MAINTAIN C-SPINE IMMOBILIZATION while undressing patient.
   ▲ if patient is potentially unstable, cut clothes from patient.
   ▲ provide for patient's privacy and warmth.
8. Quickly evaluate the possibility of transferring the patient to a trauma center and arrange for an appropriate transfer, following hospital policy.

▶ **CHEST PAIN**

▶ *Facts*

▲ More than 57 million Americans have some sort of cardiovascular disease.
▲ Annually, 1.1 million Americans suffer a myocardial infarction.
▲ 460,000 patients die each year from myocardial infarction.
▲ At least 230,000 Americans annually die **within 1 hour** of the onset of chest pain.

Assessment

A. Obtain and record triage assessment that includes:
  1. Description of pain (Table 2–5)
     ▲ **P**rovoking factors (what makes it better or worse?)
     ▲ **Q**uality of pain
     ▲ **R**egion/radiation of pain
     ▲ **S**everity of pain (1–10 scale)
     ▲ **T**ime (onset, duration, constant/intermittent)
     ▲ **T**reatment (what has the patient already tried?)
  2. Associated signs and symptoms including (see Table 2–5):
     ▲ dyspnea
     ▲ left shoulder pain
     ▲ left arm pain
     ▲ syncope
     ▲ palpitations
     ▲ fatigue
     ▲ nausea
     ▲ diaphoresis
     ▲ jaw pain
     ▲ indigestion
     ▲ dizziness
     ▲ cough
     ▲ hemoptysis
     ▲ headache
     ▲ vomiting
     ▲ behavioral changes
     ▲ back pain
  3. Associated risk factors
     ▲ atherosclerosis
     ▲ hypertension
     ▲ smoking
     ▲ diabetes
     ▲ obesity
     ▲ stress
     ▲ high cholesterol levels
     ▲ chemical dependency
     ▲ alcoholism
     ▲ lack of exercise
     ▲ cardiac surgery
     ▲ use of Viagra or herbal alternatives

Immediate Care If

▲ Male >30 years old
▲ Female >35 years old
▲ History of:
  • angina
  • myocardial infarction
• thrombolytics
• any associated risk factors
• stroke
• coronary artery disease
• cocaine use within the past 24 hours

TABLE 2–5 • Chest Pain: Causes and Characteristics

System	Cause	Characteristics
Cardiovascular	Acute myocardial infarction	• Pain may be described as aching, pressure, squeezing, burning, tightness • Intensity: vague to severe • Location of pain may be substernal, epigastric, between the shoulder blades • Radiation of the pain to the neck, jaw, arm, back • Woman may describe symptoms more of nausea, fatigue, shortness of breath • Diabetic neuropathy patients may have only vague pain
	Aneurysm	• Pain may be described as searing, continuous, severe • Radiation of pain to the back, neck, or shoulder(s) • Associated signs and symptoms: hypotension, diaphoresis, syncope
	Angina	• Pain may be described as squeezing, pressure, tightness–relieved with rest or nitroglycerin • Pain may be persistent or intermittent • Occurs with activity, anxiety, sex, heavy meals, smoking, or at rest • Associated signs and symptoms: dyspnea, nausea, vomiting, diaphoresis, indigestion
	Cardiac contusion	• Cardiac compression between the sternum and vertebral column (falls, MVAs, blunt chest trauma, etc). • May have ECG changes such as right bundle branch block, ST-T wave abnormalities, Q waves, atrial fibrillation, premature ventricular contractions, and A-V conduction disturbances
	Heart transplant	• **Rejection** may present with low-grade fever, fatigue, dyspnea, peripheral edema, pulmonary crackles, malaise, pericardial friction rub, arrhythmias, decreased ECG voltage, hypotension, increased jugular distention • **Infection** may be masked by use of immunosuppressive therapy—look for low-grade fever, cough and malaise • **Coronary heart disease** is common in patients with heart transplants
	Pericarditis	• Pain may be described as severe, continuous, worse when lying on left side • Radiation of pain to shoulder or neck • History may include recent cardiac surgery, viral illness, or myocardial infarction • Diffuse ST elevation in multiple leads • PQ segment depression
	Tachy-dysrhythmias	• Pain may be described as severe, crushing, or generalized pain over chest • Associated signs and symptoms: anxiety, tachycardia, dizziness, impending doom
Gastrointestinal	Hiatal hernia	• Pain may be described as sharp, over the epigastrium • Occurs with heavy meals, bending over, lying down
	GERD	• Pain may be described as burning, heartburn, pressure • Nonradiating pain, not influenced by activity
Musculoskeletal	Costochondritis	• Pain may be described as sharp or severe • Localized to affected area with tenderness on palpation • Associated signs and symptoms: cough, "cold"
	Muscle strain	• Pain may be described as aching • Occurs with increased use or exercise of upper-body muscles

TABLE 2–5 • Chest Pain: Causes and Characteristics (Continued)

System	Cause	Characteristics
Musculoskeletal *(continued)*		• Pain is severe, with localization over area of trauma • Pain worsens with palpations, movement, or cough • May have dyspnea
Pulmonary	Noxious fumes/smoke inhalation	• Pain may be described as searing, sense of suffocation • History includes exposure to fire, pesticide, carbon monoxide, paint, chemicals • Associated signs and symptoms: dyspnea, hypoxia, cough, pallor, ashen skin, cyanosis, singed nasal hairs, soot in oropharynx, gray or black sputum, hoarseness, drooling • Carbon monoxide poisoning may additionally show nausea, headache, confusion, dizziness, irritability, decreased judgment, ataxia, collapse
	Pleural effusion	• May be described as sharp, localized, gradual onset yet pain is continuous • Dyspnea on exertion or at rest • Pain worsens with breathing, coughing, movement • Common in smokers
	Pneumonia	• Pain may be described as continuous dull discomfort to severe pain • Associated signs and symptoms: fever, shortness of breath, tachycardia, malaise, cough, tachypnea • Children may complain of *abdominal* pain instead of chest pain
	Pneumothorax	• Pain may be described as sudden onset, sharp, severe • Associated signs and symptoms: shortness of breath
	Pulmonary embolism	• Acute shortness of breath • Risk factors include recent long-bone fractures, surgery, smoking, use of oral contraceptives, sitting for long periods of time (e.g., long air travel)
Other	Anxiety	• Pain may be described as aching, stabbing • Associated with stressful event, anxiety • Associated signs and symptoms include hyperventilation, carpal spasms, palpitations, weakness, fear, or sense of impending doom

(Hoiting, 2000; Rosen, 1999; Zavotsky, 2001)

 Interventions

1. Continue triage assessment while beginning treatment. Obtain vital signs, including:
   ▲ blood pressure
   ▲ apical heart rate
   ▲ respiratory rate
   ▲ temperature
   ▲ room air oximetry
2. Administer oxygen at 2L to 4L/minute with nasal cannula.
   Exception: Use 100% oxygen if:

   ▲ patient is obviously hypoxic
   ▲ room air oximetry is <92%
3. Obtain 12-lead ECG.
4. Continue triage if noncardiac chest pain:
   ▲ obtain basic triage assessment per protocol
   ▲ consider other sources of pain, including:
     • respiratory
     • gastrointestinal
     • musculoskeletal

► DIFFICULTY BREATHING

Assessment

A. Obtain and record triage assessment:
   1. Ask patient the time of onset of respiratory difficulty.
   2. Ask patient to identify the:
      ▲ last peak flow measurement reading (Box 2–1; Fig. 2–2)

■ Box 2–1: PEAK FLOW MEASUREMENT

Many indicators are assessed during the evaluation and treatment of patients with respiratory difficulty. Measurement of the patient's peak end-expiratory flow volume may be useful in establishing the severity of the patient's crisis and is helpful in providing a baseline understanding of the patient's respiratory status.

Peak flow readings are usually performed on patients during their initial assessment and after each nebulizer treatment. This process may be individualized to meet the treating physician's preference or the patient's ability to comply.

Asthmatic patients may be quite comfortable with the use of a peak flow meter, and many test their own peak flow at home.

Known asthmatic patients may be most familiar with color-coded peak flow readings. These are based on the individual patient's "personal best" and the recommendation of the patient's primary care physician.

COLOR CODES

The triage nurse should be aware of the following peak flow readings and the associated "color code":

GREEN ZONE: Is considered a good reading for that specific patient

YELLOW ZONE: Caution should be taken. This patient may need to have the medication regimen changed and should be in close contact with primary care physician.

RED ZONE: The patient is having frequent problems that cause concern. This patient needs to call his or her doctor immediately or go to the closest ED.

INSTRUCTIONS FOR USE OF THE PEAK FLOW METER

1. It is preferable to perform this test while the patient is standing. If the patient's condition does not permit this, then all peak flow measurements during this ED visit should be done with the patient in the same position.
2. Have the patient hold the peak flow meter lightly, making sure the fingers do not obstruct the slot or interfere with the movement of the marker.
3. Place the indicator marker at the base of the numbered scale.
4. Have the patient take in as deep a breath as possible.
5. Place the mouthpiece in the patient's mouth, and instruct him or her to seal the lips firmly around the outside of the mouthpiece.
6. Have the patient blow out as hard and as fast as possible into the mouthpiece. This action is best described as a hard "huff."
7. The indicator marker will move up the scale. Read the value.
8. Return the indicator marker to the lower end of the scale.
9. Repeat the test twice more, and document the best of the three readings.

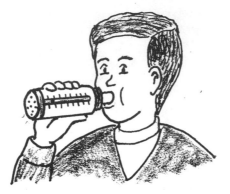

Figure 2–2. Peak flow measurement.

    ▲ date and time of the last peak flow measurement
    ▲ average peak flow reading (Tables 2–6 through Table 2–8)
3. Ask patient to rate his or her current dyspnea.
    ▲ Consider using the Modified Borg Scale (Table 2–9)
4. Assess vital signs for:
    ▲ tachypnea
    ▲ tachycardia
    ▲ bradypnea
    ▲ room air oximetry (<90% critical)
5. Assess for exertional effects due to walking or speaking in full sentences.
6. Determine associated signs and symptoms:
    ▲ pallor
    ▲ stridor

TABLE 2–6 • Predicted Average Peak Expiratory Flow (L/min): Pediatric Patients

Height (Inches)	Values (Male or Female)
44	160
46	187
48	214
50	240
52	267
54	293
56	320
58	347
60	373
62	400
64	427
66	454

TABLE 2-7 • Predicted Average Peak Expiratory Flow (L/min): Males

Age	Height (Inches)				
	60	65	70	75	80
20	554	602	649	693	740
25	543	590	636	679	725
30	532	577	622	664	710
35	521	565	609	651	695
40	509	552	596	636	680
45	498	540	583	622	665
50	486	527	569	607	649
55	475	545	556	593	634
60	463	502	542	578	618
65	452	490	529	564	603
70	440	477	515	550	587

- ▲ wheezing
- ▲ cyanosis
- ▲ retractions
- ▲ ashen skin
- ▲ crackles
- ▲ diminished breath sounds
- ▲ nasal flaring in infants
- ▲ use of accessory muscles

7. Correlate assessment finding to determine severity of asthma attack or airflow compromise (Table 2–10).
8. Place patient in respiratory isolation room when presenting with any combination of the following:
   - ▲ hemoptysis
   - ▲ fever

TABLE 2-8 • Predicted Average Peak Expiratory Flow (L/min): Females

Age	Height (Inches)				
	55	60	65	70	75
20	390	423	460	496	529
25	385	418	454	490	523
30	380	413	448	483	516
35	375	408	442	476	509
40	370	402	436	470	502
45	365	397	430	464	495
50	360	391	424	457	448
55	355	386	418	451	482
60	350	380	412	445	475
65	345	375	406	439	468
70	340	369	400	432	461

TABLE 2-9 • Dyspnea Assessment: Modified Borg Scale

Scale	Severity
0	No dyspnea at all
0.5	Very, very slight dyspnea (just barely noticeable)
1	Very slight dyspnea
2	Slight dyspnea
3	Moderate dyspnea
4	Somewhat severe dyspnea
5	Severe dyspnea
6	
7	Very severe dyspnea
8	
9	Very, very severe dyspnea
10	Maximal dyspnea

▲ night sweats
▲ profound fatigue
▲ cough lasting longer than 3 weeks
▲ significant weight loss for no apparent reason
▲ known tuberculosis (TB) history without completed treatment

9. Obtain past medical history, including any previous pulmonary diseases or injuries.

TABLE 2-10 • Severity of Asthma Attacks

Signs and Symptoms	Mild Exacerbation	Moderate Exacerbation	Severe Exacerbation	Imminent Respiratory Arrest
Short of breath	While walking	While talking (infants: have difficulty feeding)	While at rest (infants: refuse to feed)	
Position of comfort	Can lie down	Sitting	Sits up straight	
Talks in	Sentences	Phrases	Words	
Mental status	May be agitated	Usually agitated	Usually agitated	Drowsy, confused
Respiratory rate (adults)	Increased	Increased	Often >30/min	
Use of accessory muscles	No	Common	Usually	Paradoxical thoraco-abdominal movement
Wheeze	Moderate end expiratory	Loud throughout expiration	Usually loud inspiratory and expiratory	Absence of wheeze
Heart rate (adult)	<100/bpm	100–120/bpm	>120/bpm	Bradycardia

Immediate Care If

- ▲ Cyanotic
- ▲ Stridorous
- ▲ Drooling
- ▲ Room air oximetry <90%
- ▲ Patient is unable to speak in full sentences

Interventions

1. Assign patient to exam room according to ED protocol (acute vs. nonacute bed).
2. Initiate care as per protocol:
   - ▲ assist patient to undress fully.
   - ▲ place adult patients on cardiac monitor.
   - ▲ administer oxygen by 50% mask or greater.
     - • use with care if history of COPD
   - ▲ obtain initial, or repeat triage vital signs.
   - ▲ consider saline lock or normal saline IV at KVO rate per ED protocol.
   - ▲ consider drawing lab samples per ED protocol.
3. Notify ED physician of patient status.
4. Utilize appropriate flow sheet for **documentation** purposes, as necessary.

▶ DOMESTIC VIOLENCE, CHILD ABUSE, AND ELDER ABUSE

Domestic violence includes all instances of violent behavior toward persons living permanently or frequently within the same household and the abuse or neglect of children or elders.

 Assessment

A. Perform basic triage assessment per protocol.
B. Identify and document possibility or reality of domestic violence, elder abuse or neglect, or child abuse or neglect. (See Box 2–2, Documentation of Pediatric and Elder Injuries)
   1. Patient admits to history of injury by family member or friend
   2. History conflicts or is inconsistent with injuries
   3. Suspicion of domestic violence raised by emergency medical services or other third party
   4. Known previous history of domestic violence
   5. Unexplained delay in seeking treatment
   6. Patient fearful of household member or reluctant to respond when questioned
   7. Patient exhibits poor personal hygiene and/or inappropriate clothing
   8. Household member:
      ▲ over solicitous
      ▲ angry or indifferent toward patient
      ▲ prevents the patient from interacting privately or speaking openly
      ▲ refuses to provide necessary assistance
      ▲ refuses or hesitates to permit transfer to hospital
      ▲ is concerned about minor patient problem but not with the patient's serious health issue(s)
   9. Patient exhibits injuries suggestive of nonaccidental etiology:
      ▲ cigarette or other burns
      ▲ strap marks
      ▲ multiple bruises (Table 2–11)
      ▲ human bite marks

TABLE 2–11 • Bruise Assessment

Color of Bruise	Age of Bruise
Red Reddish blue	Less than 24 hours since time of injury
Dark blue Dark purple	1–4 days
Green Yellow-green	5–7 days
Yellow Brown	7–10 days
Normal tint Disappearance of bruise	1–3 weeks

> **! ALERT** For all pediatric and elderly patients who present with *any* injury, appropriate assessment for the possibility of abuse or neglect should occur. Consider an easy documentation tool, such as the sample Pediatric Injury Assessment form or the Elder Abuse form.

       ▲ long bone fractures in infants and young children

       ▲ injuries involving cheeks, ears, torso, buttocks, genitalia

  10. Parents leave injured or sick child alone in ED while they:

       ▲ go to the cafeteria

       ▲ have a cigarette

       ▲ use the telephone

C. If triage nurse suspects the possibility of domestic violence, arrange to interview patient privately and consider asking:

  1. "Have you ever been hit, slapped, kicked, or otherwise physically hurt by someone close to you?"

       ▲ If the answer is *yes,* ask the date of the last episode.

  2. "Have you ever been forced to have sexual activities?"

       ▲ If the answer is *yes,* ask the date of the last episode.

  3. If the triage nurse suspects the possibility of child or elder abuse, ask the parents or caretaker at various times throughout the patient's stay in the ED:

       ▲ "Tell me again, how did this happen?"

         • ED staff will often be able to pick up inconsistencies in the history if abuse has occurred

D. Complete remainder of basic triage assessment per protocol.

■ Box 2–2: DOCUMENTATION OF PEDIATRIC AND ELDER INJURIES

Nurses must always be alert for the possibility of abuse or neglect when triaging. Because a busy nurse can easily overlook subtle abuse injuries, departments should have a system in place that ensures that each injury suffered by a patient is adequately evaluated for the possibility of abuse or neglect.

    The following pages are sample documentation tools that have been created specifically for use in the triage setting and can be accurately completed in a matter of seconds. This provides appropriate evaluation of each patient situation as well as proper documentation of the assessment. If after completing this quick evaluation tool abuse is suspected, a more comprehensive tool on the back of the form can be used for an in-depth assessment and documentation of this child and follow-up.

INSTRUCTIONS FOR USING THE FORM

1. Fill out the demographic information on the top. For departments that use address-o-graph machines, a space has been provided at the upper right of the form.
2. While obtaining the triage history, the nurse will check off the appropriate answer for each of the boxed questions. For most nonabuse-type injuries, each answer will be "no."
3. If an answer is "yes," a clarifying comment must be made in the box to the right.
4. If suspicion of child abuse is present upon completing the front of the form, the health care team should proceed to the back of the form as necessary.
5. This form should be used as a complement to the regular departmental documentation tools, not instead of them.

PATIENT NAME _____

Pediatric Injury Assessment Form

FOR USE IN ALL CHILDREN YOUNGER THAN 18 YEARS OF AGE WITH:

- ◆ **INJURIES**
- ◆ **EXPOSURES**
- ◆ **SUSPICIOUS ILLNESSES**

DATE: _____ CHILD'S AGE: _____

WHERE DID INJURY OCCUR? _____

HISTORY PROVIDED BY: _____

HISTORY OF EVENT: _____

PERSON(S) SUPERVISING CHILD WHEN EVENT OCCURRED: _____

HIGH RISK INDICATORS FOR POSSIBLE CHILD ABUSE/NEGLECT	YES	NO	N/A	COMMENTS
Are findings inconsistent with history based on age and development of child?				
Did caretaker delay in obtaining medical care?				
Was there an unexplained absence of supervision at the time of injury?				
Is the appearance/hygiene of parent(s) inappropriate for circumstances?				
Is behavior of child inappropriate?				
Is there evidence of substance abuse?				
Is the injury a suspicious burn or human bite?				
Are there any signs of shaken baby syndrome?				
Does the injury involve the cheeks, ears, neck, chest, back, abdomen, buttocks, or genitalia?				
Are there any long bone fractures?				
Are there inconsistencies or changes in the history?				

If the answer to any of the above questions is "yes," explain under "comments."

If suspicion of child abuse for these or any other reasons exist, proceed to the back of this sheet.

Signatures _____ RN _____ MD

(over)

DESCRIPTION OF INJURY(S)							
INJURY NUMBER	TYPE OF INJURY	SHAPE	SIZE	COLOR	ESTIMATED AGE OF INJURY	STATED AGE OF INJURY	EXPLANATION BY MOTHER, FATHER, CHILD, BABY-SITTER, OTHER
1							
2							
3							
4							
5							

The investigation of child abuse may include contact with the following individuals/agencies:

1. Pediatrician _____ _____ _____
   NAME · TIME CONTACTED · COMMENTS

2. Child Protective Services _____ _____ _____
   NAME · TIME CONTACTED · COMMENTS

3. Law Enforcement
   Must be contacted if immediate intervention is needed _____ _____ _____
   AGENCY · TIME CONTACTED · COMMENTS

4. Child Abuse Hotline _____ _____ _____
   AGENCY · TIME CONTACTED · COMMENTS

5. Photographs Taken?   Yes ☐   No ☐

6. Was Child Admitted?   Yes ☐   No ☐

7. If child was not admitted, describe disposition: _____
   _____
   _____

Signatures _____ RN _____ MD

PATIENT NAME _____

Elder Abuse Assessment Form

FOR USE WITH ANY ELDER PERSON PRESENTING WITH:
- **INJURIES**
- **EXPOSURES**
- **SUSPICIOUS ILLNESSES**

DATE: _____   PATIENT'S AGE: _____

HISTORY PROVIDED BY: _____

HISTORY OF EVENT: _____

PERSON(S) WITH PATIENT WHEN EVENT OCCURRED: _____

NORMAL BEHAVIORS OF PATIENT ☐ confused   ☐ aggressive   ☐ memory loss
                              ☐ disoriented ☐ wandering   ☐ altered judgment

HIGH RISK INDICATORS FOR POSSIBLE ELDER ABUSE/NEGLECT	YES	NO	N/A	COMMENTS
Are findings inconsistent with history?				
Did patient/caretaker delay in obtaining medical care?				
Is the appearance/hygiene of patient inappropriate for circumstances?				
Is behavior of patient/caretaker inappropriate?				
Any unusual bruising patterns?				
Is the injury a suspicious burn or human bite?				
Does the injury involve the cheeks, ears, neck, chest, back, abdomen, buttocks, genitalia, wrists, or ankles?				
Is there evidence of failure to provide food, clothing, shelter, medications, supervision, etc.?				
Is there evidence of verbal, mental, sexual, financial, or substance abuse?				
Are there inconsistencies or changes in the history?				

If the answer to any of the above questions is "yes," explain under "comments."

If suspicion of **elder abuse** for these or any other reasons exist,
proceed to the back of this sheet.

Signatures _____ RN _____ MD

(over)

			DESCRIPTION OF INJURY(S)					
INJURY NUMBER	TYPE OF INJURY	SHAPE	SIZE	COLOR	ESTIMATED AGE OF INJURY	STATED AGE OF INJURY	EXPLANATION GIVEN BY	
1								
2								
3								
4								
5								

The investigation of elder abuse may include contact with the following individuals/agencies:

1. Primary Care Provider _____   _____   _____
                                NAME   TIME CONTACTED   COMMENTS

2. Adult Protective Services _____   _____   _____
                                NAME   TIME CONTACTED   COMMENTS

3. Law Enforcement _____   _____   _____
   Must be contacted if   AGENCY   TIME CONTACTED   COMMENTS
   immediate intervention is
   needed

4. Photographs Taken? Yes ☐ No ☐

5. Was Patient Admitted? Yes ☐ No ☐

6. If Patient was not admitted, describe disposition: _____
   _____

7. Comments: _____
   _____

Signatures _____ RN _____ MD

Immediate Care If

▲ Patient has serious injuries or is in danger.
- Separate the adult patient from family/care taker/significant other if possibility of assault, abuse, or neglect occurred.
- Contact social worker if one is available.

! ALERT

Refer to your department's policy for specific procedural information regarding the notification of:
- ▲ law enforcement agency
- ▲ child abuse hotline
- ▲ adult protective agency
- ▲ rape crisis advocate
- ▲ SANE or SAFE nurse

Carefully document:
- ▲ triage assessment
- ▲ detailed history/indication of any information related to the possibility of:
  - domestic violence
  - elder abuse/neglect
  - child abuse/neglect
- ▲ only that information that is pertinent to the *nursing/medical treatment* of the patient

Do NOT attempt to document for the *legal treatment* of your patient. That should be left to the law enforcement agency and the district attorney's office.

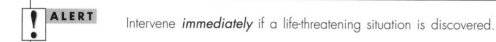

ENDOCRINE EMERGENCIES

The endocrine system is a complex one that works closely with other regulatory systems of the body. It is composed of many secretory glands, with the primary function of maintaining homeostasis within the body and regulating metabolism.

 Assessment

A. Perform basic triage assessment per protocol.

> ❗ **ALERT**   Intervene *immediately* if a life-threatening situation is discovered.

Hypoglycemia

Serum glucose <50 mg/dl in adults, <60 mg/dl in children

 Assessment

1. Common signs:
   - ▲ tachycardia
   - ▲ restlessness
   - ▲ palpitations
   - ▲ cool, diaphoretic skin
   - ▲ anxiety
   - ▲ tremors
   - ▲ irritability
2. Neurologic deficit signs:
   - ▲ headache
   - ▲ slurred speech
   - ▲ diplopia
   - ▲ seizures
   - ▲ confusion
   - ▲ combativeness
   - ▲ blurred vision
   - ▲ coma

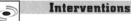 **Interventions**

1. Administer oral glucose to adult who is awake, alert, and has a gag reflex.
2. Administer 50 to 100 cc of 50% dextrose IV push to adult who is semiconscious/nonresponsive.
3. Administer 1 to 2 mg/kg of 25% dextrose IV push to child who is unconscious.

> ❗ **ALERT**   *Never* use 50% dextrose for children since it will cause vein necrosis.

▶ *Diabetic Ketoacidosis (DKA)*

 Assessment

1. Gradual onset (3–7 days) of symptoms:
   - ▲ polyuria
   - ▲ polydipsia
   - ▲ weakness
   - ▲ polyphagia
   - ▲ vomiting
   - ▲ fever
   - ▲ lethargy
   - ▲ abdominal pain
2. Objective signs:
   - ▲ hypotension
   - ▲ tachycardia
   - ▲ acetone breath
   - ▲ decreased mental status
   - ▲ Kussmaul's breathing
   - ▲ hot, dry skin with poor turgor
3. Laboratory values:
   - ▲ serum glucose >300 mg/dl
   - ▲ decreased serum bicarbonate
   - ▲ elevated acetone level
   - ▲ decreased arterial pH
   - ▲ elevated blood urea nitrogen (BUN) and creatinine
   - ▲ elevated hemoglobin and hematocrit
   - ▲ potassium level quickly fluctuates as treatment progresses

 Interventions

1. Rapidly identify DKA.
2. Continually reassess and treat with fluids, electrolytes, and insulin administration.

▶ *Hyperglycemic Hyperosmolar Nonketotic Coma (HHNC)*

- ▲ Occurs with type 2 diabetics
- ▲ History of impaired renal, cardiac, or cerebral function

Assessment

1. Slow onset (10–14 days) of symptoms:
   - ▲ polyuria
   - ▲ polydipsia
   - ▲ fever
2. Objective signs:
   - ▲ tachycardia
   - ▲ aphasia
   - ▲ hypotension
   - ▲ tremors
   - ▲ hyperreflexia
   - ▲ severe dehydration
   - ▲ decreased mental status
   - • from confused to unresponsive
   - ▲ nuchal rigidity
   - • focal seizures
3. Laboratory values:
   - ▲ serum glucose >800–1000 mg/dl
   - ▲ serum osmolality >350 mOsm/kg
   - ▲ decreased serum sodium level
   - ▲ decreased potassium level
   - ▲ elevated BUN
   - ▲ elevated hematocrit
   - ▲ elevated creatinine

Interventions

1. Maintain ABCs.
2. Continually monitor vital signs and fluid status carefully and precisely.
3. Replace fluid deficit slowly to prevent cerebral edema (may be 8–12 L).
4. Closely monitor and correct electrolyte imbalances.

Adrenal Gland Emergency: Addisonian Crisis

Assessment

1. Common signs:
   - ▲ nausea
   - ▲ vomiting
   - ▲ weakness
   - ▲ lethargy
   - ▲ hyperpigmentation
   - ▲ hypotension (not responsive to IV fluid bolus)
   - ▲ fatigue
   - ▲ anorexia
   - ▲ weight loss
   - ▲ abdominal pain
2. Less common signs:
   - ▲ diarrhea
   - ▲ delirium
   - ▲ constipation
   - ▲ increased motor activity

Interventions

1. Continually monitor cardiovascular and fluid volume status carefully.
2. Correct fluid volume deficit (usually about 3L). Aggressive replacement of fluid is necessary.
3. Administer corticosteroids, as necessary.
4. Correct hypoglycemia, as indicated.

► EYE INJURIES

Assessment

A. Obtain and record triage assessment that includes:
 1. Onset of problem (acute vs. gradual)
 2. Known precipitating event (exposure to splash or fumes, head injury, etc.)
   ▲ Was protective eyewear being worn?
   ▲ When was the injury?
   ▲ Was any care given at time of injury (rinse, patch, etc.)?
 3. Appearance of both eyes
   ▲ infection (pain, discharge, redness, edema, periorbital warmth)
   ▲ foreign body

■ Box 2–3: SNELLEN CHART FOR VISUAL ACUITY

The purpose of using the Snellen eye chart when triaging is to assess any changes in the patient's normal vision. If the patient normally wears corrective lenses for distance, then he or she should wear them during the assessment of visual acuity.

Testing for visual acuity *must* be done both before and after treatment of the patient's eye problem. This illustrates the patient's baseline on arriving to the ED and also reassesses the patient's acuity after the treatment is complete to document any improvement and to show that no harm was done by the treatment.

The results of this test are documented in the form of a fraction. The numerator is the distance the patient is standing from the chart (20 feet). The denominator, which is listed by each line of the chart, represents the distance at which the average eye can read that particular line of the chart.

TO PERFORM A VISUAL ACUITY TEST

1. Have the patient stand 20 feet away from the Snellen chart.
2. Instruct the patient to cover the *unaffected* eye.
3. Have the patient read the letters, starting at the top of the chart, using only the affected eye (you always want the patient to read with the "bad" eye first).
4. Record the last line of which the patient can read at least 50% of the letters, indicating how many were missed (e.g., right eye 20/40, −2).
5. Repeat this by covering affected eye, having the patient perform the test with the unaffected eye, and document the results.
6. Repeat this one last time, having the patient use both eyes to read the chart.

Documentation of results for the visual acuity testing should be recorded for each eye and for both eyes, should indicate if the patient used corrective lenses, and should indicate the time performed.

For example:

> 1945: with glasses:
> right eye (OD)20/30, −2
> left eye (OS)20/20, −0
> both eyes (OU)20/20, −0

    ▲ photophobic

    ▲ hyphema (blood in anterior chamber)

    ▲ deformity or irregularity of the eye

    ▲ no obvious signs of problem

  4. Visual acuity (Box 2–3)—obtain during triage assessment, and again after treatment

B. Assess blunt or sharp trauma for:

    ▲ object causing injury (tennis ball, stick, etc.)

    ▲ object size and composition

    ▲ velocity of force

    ▲ direction of force onto eye

C. Assess arc burns for:

  (Arc burns occur from unprotected exposure of the eye to welding devices.)

    ▲ time since exposure

    ▲ distance from flame

    ▲ duration of exposure

D. Assess chemical splash for:

    ▲ chemical name(s)

      • call poison control if chemical identification necessary

    ▲ initial eye symptoms/current symptoms

    ▲ irrigation substance and duration of irrigation

E. Other presentations

    ▲ central retinal artery occlusion

      • embolus/thrombus blocks the central retinal artery

      • assess for painless, unilateral loss of vision

    ▲ detached retina

      • vitreous rips from the retina and leaking fluid lifts the retina off the back of the eye

      • assess for flashing lights, floaters, a gray curtain across part of the visual field

    ▲ glaucoma

      • damage to the optic nerve from increased pressure; leading cause of blindness

      • assess for blurred vision, severe eye pain, headache, halos around lights, nausea, vomiting

    ▲ periorbital cellulitis

      • inflammatory or infectious process of the tissues anterior to the orbital septum

      • assess for erythema, warmth, tenderness, swelling, unilateral location

Immediate Care If

▲ Penetrating injury to the eye

▲ Chemical splash injury

▲ Acute, painless, unilateral loss of vision

  • Central retinal artery occlusion will cause irreversible blindness in only 30 to 60 minutes

Interventions

1. If in a penetrating injury, the foreign body is visible:

    ▲ stabilize the area surrounding the object

    ▲ avoid any movement of, or contact with, the foreign body

2. If in a penetrating injury, the foreign body is already removed, place a dry sterile patch over the eye and review patient status with the ED physician.
3. With a chemical splash injury:
    ▲ alkali is worse than acid
    ▲ test pH of eye
    ▲ review patient status with ED physician
    ▲ prepare for:
        • possible instillation of two drops of eye anesthetic in affected eye
        • flush upper and lower conjunctival fornix with direct stream of 1000 cc normal saline
4. If central retinal artery occlusion:
    ▲ ocular massage
    ▲ carbogen therapy (95% oxygen, 5% carbon dioxide) for 10 minutes every 2 hours
5. Complete remainder of basic triage assessment per protocol, and carefully document all information obtained during the triage assessment.

 ALERT Patients with eye injuries may have visual difficulties, especially depth perception. Protect for their safety while walking, and use side rails when they are in bed. Continual patient education is crucial to allay heightened patient anxiety.

FACIAL, DENTAL, AND EAR/NOSE/THROAT (ENT) INJURIES

> **! ALERT** Verify airway patency prior to and along with the assessment of these injuries. Consider possibility of c-spine or brain injury.

 Assessment

A. Obtain and record triage assessment that includes:
   ▲ nature of injury:
   - blunt
   - burn
   - blast
   - brush
   - penetrating
   ▲ mechanism of injury:
   - size
   - direction
   - velocity
   ▲ contributing factors:
   - caliber of weapon
   - height of fall
   - damage to car
   ▲ time of injury
   ▲ pain:
   - quality
   - location
   ▲ paresthesia
   ▲ immediate care of injured area
B. Utilize universal precautions during assessment progression
   ▲ face:
   - skin integrity
   - bleeding
   - wound size
   - soft tissue swelling
   - wound location
   ▲ scalp:
   - inspect and palpate for deformities or wounds
   ▲ facial structures:
   - symmetry
   - elongation of midface

- depression of bony structures
- downward displacement of globe of eye

▲ visual acuity:
  - perform for any injury involving the eye(s) or adjacent areas

▲ palpate zygomas and bony orbits:
  - swelling
  - deformity
  - point tenderness

▲ ear and mastoid areas:
  - lacerations
  - drainage
  - ecchymosis (Battle's sign)

▲ nose:
  - alignment
  - septal hematoma
  - deformity
  - epistaxis
  - swelling

▲ maxilla:
  - pain
  - ecchymosis
  - malocclusion
  - periorbital swelling
  - midface mobility

▲ teeth: using gloved finger, palpate for:
  - fractures
  - subluxations
  - avulsions

▲ jaw occlusion (bite):
  - pain
  - malalignment
  - range of motion

C. Complete remainder of triage protocol and document carefully. Up to 25% of all significant facial injuries eventually result in litigation. Consider drawings and photographs for the medical record.

D. Other presentations

▲ ear pain
  - caused by infection, pressure, injury
  - assess for fever, injury, discharge, associated signs/symptoms

▲ ear, foreign body
  - beads, rocks, food products
  - insects are extremely irritating
  - assess for ruptured eardrum, drainage, pain

▲ epistaxis
  - usually an anterior bleed from trauma, dry humidity causing dry mucous membranes, nose picking, hypertension

- • assess for stable vital signs
- ▲ nose, foreign body
  - • beads, toys, food products
  - • odor and drainage from one side of nares
  - • assess for bleeding, pain, or signs of infection
- ▲ sore throat
  - • viral, bacterial, allergic
  - • assess for airway patency, "kissing tonsils," signs of infection, ability to swallow own saliva, and pain
- ▲ toothache
  - • trauma, poor dentition, infection
  - • assess for pain and infection

Interventions

1. Continue to assess the airway patency, because the patient is at risk of developing airway compromise due to:
   - ▲ nasal and intraoral bleeding
   - ▲ fractured teeth
   - ▲ vomitus
   - ▲ secretions
   - ▲ pharyngeal hematomas
   - ▲ tongue displacement
   - ▲ edema
   - ▲ foreign bodies
   - ▲ altered level of conciousness
2. Apply ice to facial injury to minimize swelling.
3. Avulsed teeth should be:
   - ▲ handled by the crown only
   - ▲ placed in normal saline, milk, or saliva until reimplantation occurs
   - ▲ Sav-A-Tooth is an acceptable preservative and is sold over the counter (OTC)
4. Administer dT per departmental protocol.
5. Perform Halo test on nasal and ear drainage, checking for CSF leak.

FEBRILE CHILD

Assessment

A. Obtain and record triage assessment:
  1. Fever
     - ▲ onset
     - ▲ duration
     - ▲ degree
     - ▲ route obtained
  2. Associated signs, symptoms and behavior
     - ▲ rash
     - ▲ cough
     - ▲ vomiting
     - ▲ irritability
     - ▲ lethargy
     - ▲ abnormal cry
     - ▲ seizures
     - ▲ change in normal behavior
     - ▲ change in urination/stooling
     - ▲ respiratory symptoms
     - ▲ localized swelling
     - ▲ erythema
     - ▲ feeding problems
     - ▲ tugging at ears
     - ▲ limping/refusal to use an extremity
  3. Use of antipyretics, including:
     - ▲ type
     - ▲ time of last dose
     - ▲ amount administered
  4. Immunization status on chart per ED protocol
B. Obtain and record vital signs.
  1. Respirations:
     - ▲ must be counted for a full 60-second period on children <1 year old
     - ▲ document if child was crying, sleeping, etc.
  2. Heart rate:
     - ▲ apical pulse on children <3 years old
       - • caution when using heart-rate reading from automatic BP machines, as they may be easily altered by patient movement
  3. Temperature:
     - ▲ follow facility policy on route of temperature
     - ▲ recommend rectal temperature on all children <5 years old with suspicion of febrile illness
  4. Room air oximetry:
     - ▲ may need assistance from respiratory therapy (critical reading <90%)

5. Blood pressure:
   ▲ obtain after all other vital signs have been obtained
   ▲ omit if child is <5 years old and patient agitation could compromise patient's condition

Immediate Care If

▲ Patient is <12 weeks of age and rectal temperature >100.4°F as recorded by ED staff or reported by parent
▲ Rectal temperature <96°F as recorded by ED staff or reported by parent
▲ Seizure, difficulty breathing, acute onset of skin rash, or any general discomfort on the part of the triage nurse

 ALERT   Notify physician immediately if any of the above occur!

Interventions

1. Undress completely, down to diaper or underpants.
2. Wrap in blanket if necessary.
3. Administer acetaminophen/ibuprofen per department protocol.
4. Administer oxygen if:
   ▲ respiratory rate elevated for age
   ▲ room air oximetry <90%

GYNECOLOGIC ISSUES

Women seek health care for a variety of reasons from an ED or urgent care setting. Many reasons involve the female reproductive system. The triage nurse must possess excellent clinical assessment skills as well as sensitivity to the psychological needs of a woman in need of gynecologic care. Women may present with any of the following:

- ▲ fever
- ▲ fatigue
- ▲ nausea
- ▲ trauma
- ▲ dysuria
- ▲ vomiting
- ▲ vaginal bleeding
- ▲ purulent vaginal discharge
- ▲ dyspareunia
- ▲ abdominal pain
- ▲ dysmenorrhea
- ▲ sexual assault

 ALERT Sexual assault survivors are assigned a high priority and are escorted directly to a private room.

General Issues

 Assessment

A. Obtain basic triage assessment per protocol.
B. Perform abdominal pain triage assessment as necessary.

Bartholinitis

Infection or inflammation of Bartholin's glands, which lie on both sides of the vagina at the base of the labia minora.

Assessment

1. Common symptoms:
   - ▲ pain (moderate to severe)
   - ▲ swelling
   - ▲ tenderness
   - ▲ cellulitis
   - ▲ erythema
   - ▲ edema
2. Laboratory values:
   - ▲ possible culture for organism

Interventions

1. Assist with incision and drainage of gland, if indicated.
2. Administer antibiotic therapy, as prescribed.
3. Provide patient education, including:
   - ▲ sitz baths three to four times a day
   - ▲ STD transmission and available precautions
   - ▲ infection or abscess may recur

▶ *Herpes Genitalis (Herpes Simplex Virus Type 2)*

Viral infection that causes lesions on the cervix, vagina, and external genitalia

Assessment

1. Common symptoms:
   - ▲ fever
   - ▲ painful lesions
   - ▲ pruritus
   - ▲ erythema
   - ▲ malaise
   - ▲ inguinal tenderness
   - ▲ dyspareunia
   - ▲ dysuria
   - ▲ lymphadenopathy
   - ▲ bleeding
   - ▲ watery discharge from vagina or urethra
2. Clinical manifestations:
   - ▲ first manifestation is the most severe and prolonged
   - ▲ lesions occur 2 to 10 days after initial exposure and last 3 to 6 weeks

▲ lesions may proceed from macules → papules → vesicles → pustules → ulcers, which may crust and heal with scars

▲ lesions usually present as multiple vesicles with a clear, shiny, or red base

▲ lesions are usually located on the:
- vagina
- perineal area
- cervix
- vulva
- buttocks
- thighs

Interventions

1. Serology for syphilis
2. Administer acyclovir (or other antiviral agents) to decrease:
   ▲ pain
   ▲ length of infection
   ▲ healing time
3. Provide patient education, including:
   ▲ complete information on herpes genitalis, including care of lesions
   ▲ STD transmission and available precautions
   ▲ HIV counseling and testing

Pelvic Inflammatory Disease (PID)

Acute or chronic infection that involves the fallopian tubes, ovaries, uterus, pelvic peritoneum, or pelvic connective tissue

Assessment

1. History:
   ▲ new sexual partner within past 2 months
   ▲ multiple sexual partners
   ▲ early onset of sexual activity
   ▲ use of intrauterine devices
   ▲ surgical procedures
2. Common signs and symptoms:
   ▲ fever
   ▲ pelvic or abdominal pain
   ▲ purulent vaginal discharge
   ▲ irregular menstrual bleeding
   ▲ dyspareunia
   ▲ dysuria or urinary frequency

▲ walking worsens abdominal pain
  • walks hunched forward
▲ cervical motion tenderness during pelvic exam
3. Laboratory values:
  ▲ elevated white blood cell count
  ▲ pregnancy test
  ▲ serology for syphilis
  ▲ elevated sedimentation rates
  ▲ cervical cultures to isolate organisms

 Interventions

1. Administer antibiotic therapy as per current recommendations.
2. Provide patient education, including:
  ▲ early signs/symptoms of PID
  ▲ STD transmission and available precautions
  ▲ treatment of partner(s)
  ▲ HIV counseling and testing

▶ *Vaginitis*

Vaginal inflammation caused by the introduction of pathogens or irritants

Assessment

1. History:
  ▲ nature of vaginal discharge
  ▲ past illnesses or STDs
  ▲ medications being used
  ▲ vaginal hygiene practices
2. Common signs and symptoms:
  ▲ dysuria
  ▲ dyspareunia
  ▲ pelvic pain
  ▲ vaginal discharge (color, character)
  ▲ perineal
    • itching
    • burning
    • irritation
    • odor
3. Types of vaginitis:
  ▲ *Simple vaginitis* (contact vaginitis)
    • caused by poor hygiene, contact allergens, foreign bodies

  - increased vaginal discharge, with itching, edema, burning, redness
  - foul odor
  - treated by discontinuance of causative agent
▲ *Bacterial vaginosis*
  - may or may not be considered a sexually transmitted disease
  - vaginal discharge with a fishy odor
  - mild vaginal irritation
▲ *Trichomonas vaginitis*
  - copious malodorous discharge, frothy and yellow-green in color
  - may have vulvar edema and/or dysuria
  - diffuse erythema of vagina
  - treated with metronidazole (Flagyl) (contraindicated in first trimester of pregnancy)
  - partner(s) must be treated with Flagyl to prevent reinfection
▲ *Candida albicans* (fungal infection)
  - caused by use of antibiotics, steroids, douches, oral contraceptives
  - frequently associated with pregnancy, obesity, diabetes mellitus, chronic illnesses
  - vaginal discharge is thick, irritating, white/yellow color, cheese-like
  - may cause itching, dysuria, burning, dyspareunia
  - treat with antifungal agents
▲ *Neissera gonorrhea*
  - mucopurulent vaginal discharge, dysuria
  - may be asymptomatic
  - cervical motion tenderness on pelvic exam
▲ *Chlamydia trachomatis*
  - most common STD
  - usually asymptomatic, or may have vaginal discharge and/or dysuria
  - mucopurulent cervicitis on exam
4. Other:
▲ *Human Papillomavirus*
  - causes condyloma acuminatum (venereal warts)
  - highly contagious STD
  - implicated in intraepithelial neoplasia of the vulva, vagina, and cervix
  - topical treatment including laser, cryotherapy, electrocautery
  - counseling and testing for syphilis, HIV, other STDs

HEADACHE

 ## Assessment

A. Obtain and record triage assessment that includes:
1. Pain characteristics
   - ▲ **P**rovoking factors (what makes it better or worse?)
   - ▲ **Q**uality of pain
   - ▲ **R**egion/Radiation
   - ▲ **S**everity of pain (1–10 scale)
   - ▲ **T**ime (onset or duration)
   - ▲ **T**reatment
2. Associated symptoms (Table 2–12)
   - ▲ fever
   - ▲ nausea
   - ▲ vomiting
   - ▲ lethargy
   - ▲ seizure
   - ▲ syncope
   - ▲ visual changes
   - ▲ personality changes
   - ▲ rash (especially petechial)
   - ▲ change in baseline vital signs
   - ▲ change in pupil size, equality, or reaction to light
3. History of:
   - ▲ trauma
   - ▲ similar headaches
   - ▲ exposure to:
     - • fumes
     - • smoke
     - • chemicals
4. Current treatment
5. Use of anticoagulants
B. Complete basic triage assessment per protocol and **document** findings carefully.

 ## Immediate Care If

- ▲ Patient states "worst headache of my life"
- ▲ Associated fever, stiff neck, or focal signs
- ▲ Acute onset of severe headache
- ▲ History of recent head trauma
- ▲ Systolic BP >180
- ▲ Diastolic BP >115

TABLE 2-12 • Headache: Common Characteristics

Headache Type	Characteristics

Cerebellar Hemorrhage	• Pain
	  • moderate to severe headache
	• Associated signs and symptoms
	  • confusion
	  • vomiting
	  • altered gait

Cluster Headaches	• Pain
	  • very painful
	  • knifelike
	  • unilateral
	  • over the eye
	• Associated signs and symptoms
	  • excessive tearing
	  • facial swelling
	  • redness of the eye
	  • diaphoresis

Increased Intracranial Pressure	• Pain
	  • usually not excruciating
	• Associated symptoms
	  • nausea or vomiting
	  • lethargy
	  • diplopia
	  • transient visual difficulty

Meningitis	• Pain
	  • mild to severe headache
	  • neck pain or stiffness
	• Associated signs and symptoms
	  • fever
	  • malaise
	  • decreased appetite
	  • irritable

Migraines	• Pain
	  • periodic, with gradual onset
	  • throbbing, severe
	  • frequently unilateral, may progress to bilateral
	  • often above the eye(s)
	• Associated signs and symptoms
	  • photophobia
	  • sensitivity to sound
	  • nausea
	  • vomiting

Sinus Headache	• Pain
	  • over the sinus areas (above the eyes, beside the nose, or over the cheekbone)
	• Associated signs and symptoms
	  • fever

TABLE 2-12 • Headache: Common Characteristics (Continued)

Headache Type	Characteristics
Sinus Headache (continued)	• nasal drainage or congestion • ear pain • tenderness, swelling, or erythema of the sinus area

Subarachnoid Hemorrhage	• Pain
	  • "worst headache of my life"
	• Associated signs and symptoms
	  • with or without transient impairment of consciousness

Tension	• Pain
	  • diffuse yet steady dull pain or pressure
	  • "bandlike" (back of head and neck, across forehead, and/or temporal areas)

▲ Warning signs of stroke
  • weakness/numbness in the face, arm, or leg
  • visual changes (especially unilateral)
    – sudden dimness
    – blurring
    – decreased visual acuity
  • speech disturbance
    – difficulty speaking
    – difficulty understanding speech
  • unexplained
    – dizziness
    – vertigo
    – decreased coordination
  • sudden, severe headache

▶ HEAT/COLD-RELATED EMERGENCIES

▶ *Heat*

 Assessment

1. Obtain and document a routine triage assessment that includes consideration of the following:
   - ▲ heat edema
     - dependent swelling noted
     - resolves after acclimation
   - ▲ heat tetany
     - carpal—pedal spasm, secondary to hyperventilation
   - ▲ heat cramps
     - cramps in heavily exercised, overworked, fatigued muscles
     - profuse sweating without salt replacement during exercise or activity, worsened by replacement of fluid by large amount of hypotonic fluids
     - signs and symptoms:
       - muscle cramps
       - nausea
       - tachycardia
     - pallor
     - diaphoresis
     - cool skin
   - ▲ heat exhaustion
     - results from fluid and electrolyte depletion after prolonged periods of activity or exercise
     - signs and symptoms
       - core temperature is <104°F
       - headache
       - thirst
       - fatigue
       - malaise
       - confusion
       - agitation
       - mild tachycardia
       - dehydration
       - tachypnea
       - nausea and vomiting
       - muscle cramps
       - orthostatic hypotension
   - ▲ heat stroke
     - life-threatening condition
     - body loses ability to maintain normal temperature
     - severe depletion of body fluids and electrolytes

- every 1.8°F increase in core body temperature results in a 13% increase in metabolism
- increased core temperature depresses CNS, cardiac, and cellular functions
- signs and symptoms
  - core body temperature >105°F
  - severe confusion/lethargy
  - coma
  - seizure
  - ataxia
  - focal deficits
  - tachycardia
  - hypotension
  - tachypnea
  - nausea and vomiting
  - diarrhea
  - dry, hot skin
  - acute renal failure
  - rhabdomyolysis
  - hepatic failure

Interventions

1. Maintain ABCs.
2. Immediate cooling of the body.
3. Supportive rehydration, as appropriate.

▶ Cold

Assessment

1. Obtain and document a routine triage assessment that includes consideration of the following:
   - ▲ frostbite, general
     - occurs with prolonged exposure to freezing, wet situations
     - penis, fingers, toes, ears, and nose are the most commonly affected areas
     - initial appearance of the injury does not predict long-term effects of the injury
     - ice crystals form and expand in the extracellular spaces if tissue temperature is less than 59°F
   - ▲ superficial frostbite
     - skin structure is only involved
     - skin initially appears to be white, waxy, and/or mottled
     - skin does not blanch
     - skin eventually appears to be hyperemic and edematous as warming occurs
     - loss of sensation to touch, pain, or temperature with frozen skin
     - stinging, numbness, burning
     - no long-term tissue loss
   - ▲ deep frostbite
     - subcutaneous, muscle, nerve and/or bone involved
     - tissue feels frozen hard
     - initially no sensation in the area

- upon warming, there is severe pain and burning sensation and development of edema
- if deep structures were damaged, there is decreased mobility even after warming
- tissue loss is inevitable
▲ hypothermia (general)
- impaired thermoregulation through
  - age-fragile patients (very young or old)
  - endocrine failure
  - malnutrition
  - central CNS conditions affecting the hypothalamus
  - immersion if cold water, cold weather, and/or wet clothing increase heat loss
  - shivering increases the metabolic rate in an attempt to raise the body temperature
▲ mild hypothermia
- body temperature 93°– 95°F (35°– 36°C)
- signs and symptoms
  - conscious
  - alert
  - shivering
  - tachycardia
  - slurred speech

  - amnesia
  - poor coordination
  - increased urine production
▲ moderate hypothermia
- body temperature is 86°– 93°F (30°– 34°C)
- signs and symptoms (Table 2–13)
  - difficulty speaking
  - absence of shivering
  - muscle rigidity
  - hyperglycemia
  - bradycardia
  - ECG changes
  - hypotension
  - decreased respiratory effort
  - renal blood flow begins to slow
▲ severe hypothermia
- body temperature falls below 86°F (<30°C) (see Table 2–13)
- signs and symptoms
  - unconscious
  - decreased renal function
  - relative central hypovolemia
  - shallow or absent respirations
  - ventricular dysrhythmias
  - cardiopulmonary arrest

TABLE 2-13 • Normal Signs and Symptoms Associated with Falling Body Temperatures

Temperature (Celsius)	Signs/Symptoms
35	Maximum shivering
34	Amnesia, dysarthria
33	Ataxia, apathy
32	Stuporous
31	Shivering stops
30	Atrial fib
28	Ventricular fib
27	Voluntary motion stops
24	Significant hypotension
19	Flat EEG
18	Asystole
15.2	Lowest accidental hypothermia survival

► HEMATOLOGIC EMERGENCIES

Typically, patients who present to the ED with hematologic emergencies have been previously diagnosed with blood disorders. They should be considered life-threatening episodes, whether they are acute events or exacerbations of a chronic disorder.

► *General Issues*

 Assessment

A. Obtain basic triage assessment per protocol.
B. For both chronic and acute presentations, assess patients for:
  1. Common symptoms:
    ▲ weakness
    ▲ syncope
    ▲ fatigue
    ▲ dizziness
    ▲ headache
    ▲ fever
    ▲ exertional dyspnea
  2. Skin changes:
    ▲ color
    ▲ texture
    ▲ petechiae
    ▲ moisture
    ▲ cyanosis
    ▲ ecchymosis
    ▲ turgor
    ▲ temperature
    ▲ jaundice
    ▲ pallor
  3. Associated factors:
    ▲ precipitating event
    ▲ bleeding tendencies
    ▲ aggravating factors
    ▲ alleviating factors
    ▲ joint or muscle
      • redness
      • swelling
      • decreased range of motion

▲ symptoms
- onset
- nature
- severity
- duration

►Sickle Cell Anemia

This occurs primarily in African Americans and persons of Mediterranean descent.

 Assessment

1. Common precipitating events:
   - ▲ infection
   - ▲ depression
   - ▲ dehydration
   - ▲ fever
   - ▲ hypoxemia
   - ▲ anxiety
   - ▲ exposure to cold environment
2. Common symptoms:
   - ▲ fever
   - ▲ erythema
   - ▲ organomegaly
   - ▲ jaundice
   - ▲ dehydration
   - ▲ inflamed joints
   - ▲ localized warmth
   - ▲ pallor
   - ▲ soft tissue swelling
   - ▲ severe, acute onset of pain
3. Laboratory values:
   - ▲ chronic anemia
   - ▲ elevated bilirubin count
   - ▲ reticulocyte count of 5% to 30%
   - ▲ variable platelet count
   - ▲ elevated white blood cell count

 Interventions

1. Maintain ABCs.
2. Administer oxygen.

3. Insert IV access for:
   - ▲ fluids
   - ▲ medications
   - ▲ blood products

▶ *Hemophilia*

This is characterized by excessive, prolonged, or delayed internal or external bleeding from inherited coagulation disorders, usually occurring in males.

Assessment

1. Hemarthroses (bleeding into the joint):
   - ▲ common sites:
     - • ankle
     - • elbow
     - • wrist
     - • knee
     - • shoulder
     - • hip
   - ▲ common signs and symptoms:
     - • pain
     - • swelling
     - • localized warmth
     - • decreased range of motion
2. Intramuscular bleeding:
   - ▲ common sites:
     - • thigh
     - • calf
     - • forearm
     - • iliopsoas (abdomen)
3. Other areas of bleeding:
   - ▲ common sites:
     - • oral cavity
     - • intracranial
     - • genitourinary
     - • gastrointestinal
4. Laboratory values:
   - ▲ normal or elevated platelet count
     - • normal or abnormal prothrombin time (PT)
     - • prolonged partial thromboplastin time (PTT)
     - • normal or abnormal bleeding time

Interventions

1. Maintain ABCs.
2. Achieve rapid hemostasis.
3. Insert IV access for:
   - ▲ fluids
   - ▲ medications
   - ▲ blood products
   - ▲ factor replacement
4. Treat affected extremity with:
   - ▲ ice
   - ▲ elevation
   - ▲ immobilization
5. Minimize number of venipunctures.
6. Always use small-gauge needles.

▶ INFECTIOUS DISEASES

It is essential for the triage nurse to maintain a confidential, nonjudgmental atmosphere when interviewing a patient. The patient may fear rejection from friends and family, as well as the perceived social stigma and isolation related to the illness.

▶ *General Issues*

 Assessment

A. Complete the basic triage assessment per protocol.
B. Perform a subjective assessment.
   1. Signs and symptoms:
      ▲ fever
      ▲ weakness
      ▲ malaise
      ▲ change in level of consciousness
      ▲ anorexia
      ▲ fatigue
      ▲ chills
      ▲ rash
      ▲ lesions or wounds
      ▲ mucopurulent discharge
   2. Specific details:
      ▲ onset of symptoms
      ▲ exacerbating factors
      ▲ rate of symptom development
      ▲ response to any self-treatment
   3. Disease or drugs that would compromise patient's immune system:
      ▲ diabetes
      ▲ hematologic pathology
      ▲ antibiotics
      ▲ cancer
      ▲ immunosuppressive drugs
      ▲ HIV/AIDS
      ▲ chemotherapy
      ▲ steroids
   4. High-risk patient populations:
      ▲ homeless
      ▲ incarcerated
      ▲ psychiatric
      ▲ sociopathic behavior

▲ alcohol or substance abuse
▲ age fragile (infant or elderly)
▲ day care centers
▲ prolonged immobility
▲ nursing homes

C. Perform an objective assessment.
  1. Neurologic findings:
     ▲ confusion
     ▲ apprehension
     ▲ lethargy
     ▲ agitation
  2. Vital signs:
     ▲ fever
     ▲ hypotension
     ▲ orthostatic vitals signs
     ▲ tachycardia
     ▲ tachypnea
  3. Ears, nose, throat, and lymph nodes:
     ▲ pain
     ▲ swelling
     ▲ discharge or exudate
     ▲ lesions
     ▲ erythema
  4. Chest:
     ▲ lung sounds
     ▲ heart sounds
     ▲ productive cough
  5. Abdomen:
     ▲ nausea/vomiting
     ▲ diarrhea
     ▲ bowel sounds
     ▲ pain on palpation
  6. Genitals:
     ▲ lesions
     ▲ parasites
     ▲ exudates
     ▲ inflammation
  7. Skin or extremities:
     ▲ petechiae
     ▲ joint pain
     ▲ lesions
     ▲ abscesses
     ▲ nuchal rigidity
     ▲ erythema
     ▲ cellulitis
     ▲ warmth
     ▲ swelling
     ▲ purpura
     ▲ tenderness
     ▲ limited range of motion

Interventions

1. Will vary with each disease or infectious process
2. Consider isolation room based on patient history and assessment of current symptoms (Table 2–14, Table 2–15, Table 2–16; Box 2–4, Box 2–5).

TABLE 2–14 • Communicable Diseases

Disease	Mode of Transmission	Incubation Period (Days)	Contagious Period (Days)
Acquired immunodeficiency syndrome (AIDS) Human immunodeficiency virus (HIV)	Blood, breast milk, body tissues, fluids exchanged during sexual contact Other body fluids: saliva, urine, tears, bronchial secretions (especially if blood is present)	Variable incubation rates Virus exposure to seroconversion (HIV+): ~1–3 months HIV+ to AIDS from <1 year to 10 years	Although unknown, it is believed to begin just after onset of HIV and extend throughout life
Botulism	Contaminated food products	Within 12–36 hours of consumption, up to several days	Not contagious from secondary person-to-person contact
Bronchiolitis	Respiratory	4–6 days	Onset of cough until 7 days
Chancroid	Direct sexual contact with open or draining lesions	3–5 days, up to 14 days	Until treated with antibiotic and lesions healed—usually about 1–2 weeks
Chickenpox (varicella)	Direct person-to-person contact Respiratory droplet	Commonly 14–16 days	1 to 5 days before the onset of the rash— until all sores have crusted over, usually 10–21 days
Chlamydia	Sexual intercourse	Approximately a minimum of 7–14 days.	Unknown
"Cold," cough, croup	Respiratory	2–5 days	Onset of runny nose and/or cough until fever is gone
Conjunctivitis Viral	Direct or indirect contact	1–12 days	4–14 days after onset of symptoms (minimally contagious)
Bacterial	Respiratory Direct contact with eye drainage	24–72 hours	Until treated with antibiotics
Fifth disease	Respiratory	Variable 4–20 days	7 days before rash develops, probably not communicable after rash starts
Giardia	Fecal contamination of food or water	3–25 days	Entire period of infection, often months
Gonorrhea	Sexual contact	2–7 days	Continues until treatment begins

TABLE 2–14 • Communicable Diseases (Continued)

Disease	Mode of Transmission	Incubation Period (Days)	Contagious Period (Days)
Hand, foot and mouth disease (Coxsackievirus)	Direct contact with nasal or throat secretions, fecal Droplet	3–6 days	Onset of mouth ulcers until fever gone— perhaps as long as several weeks with fecal contamination
Hepatitis A	Fecal–oral route Food contamination	15–50 days	During last half of incubation period until after 1st week of jaundice
Hepatitis B	Blood, saliva, semen, vaginal fluid	45–180 days	Infective many weeks before onset of first symptom, until completion of acute clinical course of infection
Hepatitis C	Blood and plasma Percutaneous exposure	2 weeks–6 months	From 1+ weeks before onset of symptoms; may persist indefinitely
Herpes simplex *Type 1*	Saliva	2–12 days	From onset of sores to 7 weeks after recovery from stomatitis
Type 2	Sexual contact (oral or genital)	2–12 days	7–12 days
Herpes (varicella) zoster (shingles)	Soiled dressings or articles	Can be 2–3 weeks	1 to 5 days before the onset of the rash— until all sores have crusted over, usually 10–21 days
Impetigo *Staph*	Hand–skin contact	4–10 days	Until draining lesions heal
Strep	Respiratory droplet Direct contact	1–3 days	Untreated: weeks— months Treated: 24 hours on antibiotics
Influenza	Airborne Direct contact	1–3 days	Children: 7 days Adults: 3–5 days
Kawasaki	Unknown Seasonal variation	Unknown	Unknown
Legionnaire pneumonia	Airborne	2–10 days	Person-to-person: none

TABLE 2–14 • Communicable Diseases (Continued)

Disease	Mode of Transmission	Incubation Period (Days)	Contagious Period (Days)
Lice			
Head/Body	Direct contact, indirect contact with objects	7–13 days Egg-to-egg cycle lasts 3 weeks	Continuous if alive, until 1st treatment Live off host for 7–21 days
Pubic (crabs)	Sexual contact		Live off host for 2 days
Lyme disease	Tickborne	3–32 days	Person-to-person: none
Measles (rubeola)	Airborne Direct contact with nasal secretions	7–18 days	Before the onset of symptoms to 4 days after the appearance of the rash
Meningitis			
Bacterial: meningococcal	Direct contact: respiratory droplet from nose and mouth	2–10 days	Usually after 24 hours on antibiotic therapy
Bacterial: haemophilus	Droplet from nose and mouth	2–4 days	Noncommunicable within 24–48 hours on antibiotic therapy
Viral	Varies with specific infectious agent		Variable, often approximately 7 days
Mononucleosis	Saliva	4–6 weeks	Prolonged, possibly a year
Pertussis	Direct contact Airborne droplet	6–20 days	Gradually decreases over 3 weeks
Pinworms	Direct transfer (anus to mouth) Indirect contact (infested bed, etc.)	2–6 weeks	As long as females are alive Eggs survive for about 2 weeks
Rabies	Saliva Direct contact (bite, scratch) Indirect contact	3–8 weeks	3–7 days before the onset of symptoms
Ringworm			
Tinea capitus (scalp)	Direct skin-to-skin Indirect contact (cloth seats, combs, etc.)	10–14 days	Viable fungus may persist on contaminated articles for long periods of time
Tinea corporis (body)	Direct or indirect contact with infected people, articles, floors, benches, animals, shower stalls	4–10 days	While lesions are present and as long as viable fungus remains on articles
Rocky Mountain spotted fever	Tickborne	3–14 days	Noncommunicable person to person Tick remains infective for life, as long as 18 months

TABLE 2–14 • Communicable Diseases (Continued)

Disease	Mode of Transmission	Incubation Period (Days)	Contagious Period (Days)
Roseola	Unknown Possibly saliva	10–15 days	Onset of fever until rash is gone
Rotavirus	Fecal–oral route Possible respiratory	24–72 hours	Average 4–6 days
Rubella	Direct contact nasal secretions Droplet	14–23 days	1 week before—to at least 4 days after onset of rash
Salmonella	Ingestion of contaminated food	6–72 hours	Throughout the course of infection
Scabies	Direct skin to skin contact	2–6 weeks	Until mites and eggs are destroyed
Scarlet fever	Large respiratory droplet Direct contact	1–3 days	Untreated: 10–21 days Treated: 24 hrs of antibiotic therapy
Shigella	Fecal–oral route Ingestion of contaminated food	12–96 hours	During acute infection until infectious agent no longer in feces (~ 4 weeks)
Sore throat *Strep*	Large respiratory droplet Direct contact	1–3 days	Untreated: 10–21 days Treated: after 24 hours of antibiotic therapy
Viral	Direct contact Inhalation of airborne droplet	1–5 days	Onset of sore throat until fever gone
Syphilis	Direct contact with moist lesions and body fluids	10 days–3 months	Untreated: variable and indefinite Treated: after 24–48 hours of antibiotic therapy
Tetanus	Spores enter open wound	3–21 days	Noncommunicable from person to person
Trichomoniasis	Sexual contact through vaginal or urethral secretions	4–24 days	Untreated: may be symptom-free carrier for years
Tuberculosis	Airborne droplet	4–12 weeks	Degree of communicability depends on many factors Treated: within a few weeks Children with TB usually not infectious

(Nettina, 1997; Bartlett, 2002)

TABLE 2-15 • "Cold" Versus Flu Symptom Comparison

Symptom	"Cold"	Flu
Fever	Rare	Usually high (102°–104°F) Lasts 3–4 days
Headache	Rare	Yes
Body aches and pains	Slight	Often severe
Fatigue	Mild	Lasts 2–3 weeks
Extreme exhaustion	No	Early in illness Lasts a few days
Stuffy or runny nose	Yes	Occasionally
Sneezing	Yes	Occasionally
Sore throat	Yes	Occasionally
Chest discomfort and/or cough	Mild-to-moderate hacking cough	Yes May be severe
Complications	Sinus congestion Ear pain	Bronchitis Pneumonia

TABLE 2-16 • Sexually Transmitted Diseases

Disease	Clinical Presentation	Complications and Long-Term Risks
AIDS/HIV	May remain asymptomatic for many years Developing sign and symptoms include: fatigue, fever, poor appetite, unexplained weight loss, generalized lymphadenopathy, persistent diarrhea, night sweats	Disease progression (from HIV to AIDS) is variable, from a few months to 12 years Early intervention is essential in preserving and maintaining optimal health status
Chancroid	Painful genital ulceration(s) with tender inguinal adenopathy Ulcers may be necrotic or erosive	Chancroid has been associated with increased risk of acquiring HIV infection Should be tested for other infections that cause ulcers (e.g. syphilis)
Chlamydial cervicitis	Yellow mucopurulent cervical exudate May or may not be symptomatic Male sexual partner will likely have nongonococcal urethritis	Untreated, may develop endometritis, salpingitis, ectopic pregnancy, and/or subsequent infertility High prevalence of coinfection with gonococcal infection Infection during pregnancy may lead to premature rupture of the membranes; pneumonia or conjunctivitis in the infant
Enteric infections	Sexually transmissible enteric infections particularly among gay men Abdominal pain, fever, diarrhea, vomiting	Occurs frequently with oral–genital and oral–anal contact Infections can be life-threatening if they become systemic Organisms may be Shigella, hepatitis A, Giardia

TABLE 2–16 • Sexually Transmitted Diseases (Continued)

Disease	Clinical Presentation	Complications and Long-Term Risks
Epididymitis	May or may not be transmitted sexually Can be asymptomic Nonsexually transmitted, is associated with a urinary tract infection Unilateral testicular pain, swelling	Usually caused by gonorrhea or chlamydia May be caused by E. coli after anal intercourse Must rule out a testicular torsion before making the diagnosis of epididymitis
Genital warts	Soft, fleshy, painless growth(s) around the anus, penis, vulvovaginal area, cervix, urethra, or perineum	Caused by the human papillomavirus Must rule out other causes of lesion(s), such as syphilis, etc. Lesions may cause tissue destruction Cervical warts are associated with neoplasia
Gonorrhea	Males may have dysuria, urinary frequency, thin clear or yellow urethral discharge Females may have mucopurulent vaginal discharge, abnormal menses, dysuria, or may be asymptomatic	Untreated, risk of arthritis, dermatitis, bactermia, meningitis, endocarditis At risk: males—epididymitis, infertility, urethral stricture, and sterility; females—pelvic inflammatory diseases; newborns—ophthalmia neonatorum, pneumonia
Hepatitis B	Anorexia, malaise, nausea, vomiting, abdominal pain, jaundice, skin rash, arthralgias, arthritis	Chronic hepatitis, cirrhosis, liver cancer, liver failure, death Chronic carrier occurs in 6–10% of cases Infants born with hepatitis B are at high risk for developing chronic liver disease
Herpes genitalis (Herpes simplex type 2)	Clustered vesicles that rupture, leaving painful, shallow genital ulcer(s) that eventually crust Initial outbreak lasts for 14–21 days, subsequent outbreaks are less severe and last 8–12 days	Other causes of genital ulcers (syphilis, chancroid, etc.) must be ruled out
Nongonococcal urethritis	Dysuria, urinary frequency, mucoid to purulent urethral discharge Some men may be asymptomatic Female sexual partners may have cervicitis or PID	Can be caused by chlamydia, mycoplasma, trichomonas, or herpes simplex Can cause urethral strictures, prostatitis, epididymitis
Pelvic inflammatory disease (PID)	Lower abdominal pain, fever, cervical motion tenderness, dyspareunia, purulent vaginal discharge, dysuria, increased abdominal pain while walking	Must rule out appendicitis or ectopic pregnancy Risk for pelvic abscess, future ectopic pregnancy, infertility, pelvic adhesions
Proctitis	Sexually transmitted GI illnesses Proctitis occurs with anal intercourse, resulting in inflammation of the rectum, with anorectal pain, tenesmus, and rectal discharge	May be caused by chlamydia, gonorrhea, herpes simplex, and syphilis Among patients coinfected with HIV, herpes proctitis may be severe
Proctocolitis	Sexually transmitted GI illnesses Proctocolitis occurs with either anal intercourse or with oral–fecal contact, resulting in symptoms of proctitis, as	May be caused by Campylobacter, Shigella, or Chlamydia Other opportunistic infections may be involved among immunosuppressed

TABLE 2-16 • Sexually Transmitted Diseases (Continued)

Disease	Clinical Presentation	Complications and Long-Term Risks
Proctocolitis (continued)	well as diarrhea, abdominal cramps, and inflammation of the colonic mucosa	HIV patients
Pubic lice	Slight discomfort to intense itching May have pruritic, erythematous macules, papules, or secondary excoriation in the genital area If lice are found on the eyelashes, they are usually pubic lice	Sexual partners within the last month should be treated May develop lymphadenitis or a secondary bacterial infection of the skin or hair follicle
Scabies	The mite burrows under the skin of the fingers, penis, and wrists Scabies among adults may be sexually transmitted, while usually *not* sexually transmitted among children Itching (worse at night), papular eruptions, and excoriation of the skin	Sexual partners, household members, and close contacts within the past month should be examined and treated May develop a secondary infection, often with nephrotogenic streptococci
Syphilis		
Primary syphilis	Painless, indurated, ulcer (chancre) at site of infection approximately 10 days to 3 months after exposure	All genital ulcers should be suspected to be syphilitic. Should be tested for HIV, and retested again in 3 months
Secondary syphilis	Rash, mucocutaneous lesions, lymphadenopathy, condylomata lata Symptoms occur 4–6 weeks after exposure and resolve spontaneously within weeks to 12 months	At-risk sex partners are those within the past 3 months plus duration of symptoms for primary syphilis, and 6 months plus duration of symptoms for secondary syphilis
Latent syphilis	Seroreactive yet asymptomatic Can be clinically latent for a period of weeks to years Latency sometimes lasts a lifetime	Should be clinically evaluated for tertiary disease (i.e., aortitis, neurosyphilis, etc.) At-risk sex partners are those within the past year for early latent syphilis
Tertiary/Late syphilis	May have cardiac, neurologic, ophthalmic, auditory, or gummatous lesions	
Neurosyphilis	May see a variety of neurologic signs and symptoms, including ataxia, bladder problems, confusion, meningitis, uveitis May be asymptomatic	Diagnosis made based on a variety of tests including: reactive serologic test results, cerebrospinal fluid (CSF) protein or cell count abnormalities, positive VDRL on CSF
Congenital syphilis	Needs to be ruled out for infants born to mothers with untreated syphilis, mothers who received incomplete treatment, or insufficient follow-up of reported treated syphilis Serologic tests for mother and infant can be negative at delivery if mother was infected late in pregnancy	Syphilis frequently causes abortion, stillbirth, and complications of prematurity of infant Treated infants must be followed very closely and retested every 2–3 months Most infants are nonreactive by 6 months Infants with positive CSF should be retested every 6 months and be retreated if still abnormal at 2 years
Trichomoniasis vaginitis	Profuse, thin, foamy, greenish-yellow discharge with foul odor May be asymptomatic Male partners may have urethritis	Trichomoniasis often coexists with gonorrhea Perform a complete STD assessment if trichomoniasis is diagnosed

(Bartlett, 2002; Lippincott, 1996; Nettina, 1997; Rosen, 1999)

■ Box 2–4: **UNIVERSAL (STANDARD) PRECAUTIONS**

The triage nurse must practice according to the guidelines of universal precautions for each and every patient who enters the department for care. It is important to remember that each patient is potentially the carrier of a contagious disease. The Occupational Safety and Health Administration (OSHA) maintains strict standards that apply to everyone who is at risk of coming into contact with blood or body fluids during the performance of routine job duties. It is up to the individual employee and each facility to know and adhere to the current standards of universal precautions.

In addition to blood, other potentially infectious materials include:

- semen
- vaginal secretions
- cerebrospinal fluid
- synovial fluid
- any body fluid visibly contaminated with blood
- any unidentifiable body fluids
- peritoneal fluid
- amniotic fluid
- breast milk
- saliva

The goal of universal precautions is to minimize or eliminate the significant health risk posed by occupational exposure to blood and other potentially infectious materials that may contain blood-borne pathogens. Among the diseases that health care workers are at risk of contracting are hepatitis B, human immunodeficiency virus (HIV), hepatitis C, syphilis, and other contagious blood-borne diseases.

Gloves, goggles, and masks should routinely be stocked in the triage room and utilized by the triage nurse. Good handwashing or the use of an approved hand disinfectant is essential between patients. Hands should always be washed immediately upon the removal of gloves.

Red-bag or biohazard trash receptacles should be available for the disposal of contaminated products and used for all potentially contaminated trash.

It is important for the triage nurse to include the patient when utilizing universal precautions and to educate the patient about the need for such special care. Patients may be anxious regarding the use of protective wear, and simple patient education can help reduce their anxiety. The triage nurse should also take a proactive role in teaching young children, who may be curious and attracted to the brightly colored biohazard receptacle, and keep them from playing with these trash cans.

■ Box 2–5: **ISOLATION**

Any patient who presents with a potentially contagious skin rash must be escorted directly from the triage room into the department's isolation room. This room may also be utilized for enteric precautions. The patient should be taught the importance of this isolation and kept from walking through the main ED whenever possible.

Any patient who presents with a potentially contagious respiratory condition should be considered for placement in the negative-pressure room (if your department has one). If the patient's condition is of high acuity, the triage nurse should decide which bed in the ED will best suit the patient's needs and maintain respiratory isolation within that examination room. The patient should wear a mask when being transported through the department or the facility hallways.

A patient presenting with chickenpox must be placed in the isolation room and be isolated for both respiratory and contact isolation.

After the discharge of a patient with a contagious illness, the room must be thoroughly decontaminated per hospital policy.

► MENTAL HEALTH

▲ A mental health emergency is any alteration in thought process, feelings, or actions for which immediate therapeutic interventions are indicated.
▲ It is essential to develop rapport quickly with the patient since this has a great impact on the nurse's
ability to accurately complete the triage assessment of him or her.

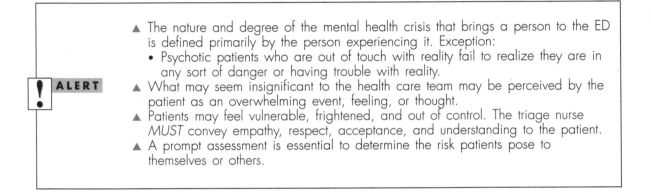

ALERT

▲ The nature and degree of the mental health crisis that brings a person to the ED
is defined primarily by the person experiencing it. Exception:
 • Psychotic patients who are out of touch with reality fail to realize they are in
 any sort of danger or having trouble with reality.
▲ What may seem insignificant to the health care team may be perceived by the
patient as an overwhelming event, feeling, or thought.
▲ Patients may feel vulnerable, frightened, and out of control. The triage nurse
MUST convey empathy, respect, acceptance, and understanding to the patient.
▲ A prompt assessment is essential to determine the risk patients pose to
themselves or others.

► *General Issues*

Assessment

A. Obtain and record complete triage assessment:
  1. Perform a basic triage assessment per protocol.
  2. Obtain a history of chief complaint.
     ▲ current symptoms, including:
       • nature
       • onset
       • duration
     ▲ in the presence of delusions or hallucinations, consider asking:
       • "Are you hearing voices?"
       • "What are the voices telling you?"
       • "Do you want to hurt yourself? Someone else?"
       • "Do you have a plan?"
       • "Did you bring anything with you?"
     ▲ recent changes:
       • life stressors
       • medication
       • sexual interest

- appetite
- sleep pattern
- digestive functioning
- level of functioning:
  - socially
  - physically
  - occupationally
  - mentally
  - academically
3. Obtain a past history.
  ▲ medical
  - head trauma
  - Alzheimer's
  - brain tumor
  - infections
  - hypoxia
  - renal failure
  - seizure disorder
  - multiple sclerosis
  - endocrine dysfunctions
  - metabolic abnormalities
  - alcohol intoxication or withdrawal
  - drug ingestion (PCP, LSD, cocaine, etc.)
  - liver failure
  - nutritional deficiencies
  - AIDS-related dementia
  ▲ psychiatric
  - anxiety
  - somatoform disorders
  - schizophrenia
  - eating disorders
  - personality disorders
  - depression
  - bipolar (manic depression)
  - self-harming behaviors
  - suicidal or homicidal behavior
  - sexual and gender identity disorders
  ▲ familial
  - substance abuse
  - domestic violence
  - mental illness among family members
  - income level
  - living arrangements
  - legal issues
  - use of nicotine

4. Perform a physical assessment.
   ▲ assess for:
   - diaphoresis
   - agitation
   - cool, clammy skin
   - tachycardia
   - thought process
   - anxiety
   - pallor
   - flushing
   - dystonic movements
   - speech irregularities
   - respiratory distress or tachypnea
   - motor restlessness or pacing
5. Perform a mental status examination.
   ▲ assess for obvious changes in behavior, speech, thought process
   ▲ refer to "Pearls of Triage Wisdom: Mental Health" (later in this book) for a complete description of how to perform a mental status exam.
6. Consider the patient's age.
   ▲ pediatric or adolescent
   - age-appropriate behaviors vary.
   - differentiation between abnormal behavior and normal adjustment behavior is difficult.
   - assess for:
     - extreme sadness
     - overreacts frequently
     - extremely fearful
     - poor concentration
     - chemical dependency
     - drop in school grades
     - defiance of rules
     - switching friends
     - change in behavior
     - inflicts harm on others
     - persistent nightmares
     - anorexia or bulimia
     - breaks the law
     - hopelessness
     - constant or extreme anger
     - cries easily for "no reason"
     - desires to be alone constantly
     - possibility of abuse or assault
     - secrecy or isolation
     - emotional highs and lows
     - withdrawal from family and friends
     - drop in work or sport performance

 – focused on topics such as death
 – abuses laxatives
 – destroys property
 – performs life-threatening acts
▲ elderly
 • assess for:
 – chemical dependency
 – cognitive impairment
 – organic manifestations
 – withdrawal or isolation
 – social stressors
 – personal loss
 – thorough review of medications (prescriptions, OTC, natural or home remedies)

Interventions

1. Protect safety of patient, staff, and visitors.
   ▲ Involve security as needed or indicated per hospital protocol.
   ▲ Remove items from patient's room that may cause harm.
   ▲ Remove patient belongings from room, store safely away from patient.
   ▲ Do not allow patient to cover his or her head with a blanket.
2. Listen to patient and acknowledge statements.
3. Focus on the patient's safety and needs; work to develop rapport.
4. Avoid condescending speech, threatening movements, or any staff behavior that would further aggravate the patient.
5. Use brief, simple explanation of what you are going to do and what the expectations are during the patient's stay in ED.
6. Remove high-risk patients to a quiet yet closely monitored setting as soon as possible. These include:
   ▲ psychotic patients
   ▲ patients at risk of harming self or others
   ▲ agitated patients
   ▲ survivors of domestic violence
   ▲ confused patients
7. Remove patient clothing if a flight risk or suicidal risk
8. Consider 1:1 staff monitoring of patient on safety watch—keep patient in view at all times.

Alcohol Abuse, Alcoholism, and Alcohol Withdrawal

▲ It is estimated that 13.8 million people abuse alcohol.
 • 9.8 million males
 • 3.9 million females
▲ Approximately 43% of adults in the United States have been exposed to alcoholism within their own family.

▲ In 2000, there were 19,358 alcohol-induced deaths in the USA, not counting motor vehicle accidents (according to the CDC).

▲ Alcohol is involved in:
- 86% of homicides
- 65% of suicide completions
- 57% of men involved in marital violence
- 50% of boating fatalities
- 42% of violent crime
- 40% of industrial fatalities
- 38% of all traffic fatalities
- 37% of sexual offenses
- 27% of women involved in marital violence (CDC, 1999; NCADD, 2000; NIAAA, 1997; Varcarcolis, 1998)

The nurse should always stay alert for signs of alcohol use or abuse and carefully utilize any information gathered when assigning a triage acuity and formulating a plan of care for the patient.

 Assessment

A. Perform a general mental health assessment per protocol.
1. Associated information:
   - ▲ description of current drinking episode
   - ▲ pattern of drinking behavior
   - ▲ length of time since last drink
   - ▲ presence of poly-substance abuse
2. Physical findings or medical history of:
   - ▲ poor dentition
   - ▲ hoarseness
   - ▲ esophageal varices
   - ▲ arrhythmias
   - ▲ ascites
   - ▲ liver enlargement
   - ▲ myopathy
   - ▲ skin lesions
   - ▲ gout
   - ▲ hypoglycemia
   - ▲ delirium tremens
   - ▲ seizures
   - ▲ hepatic disease
   - ▲ ulcers/gastritis
   - ▲ cardiomyopathy
   - ▲ memory deficits
   - ▲ sleep disturbances
   - ▲ "blackouts"
   - ▲ hallucinations (usually visual or tactile)
   - ▲ frequent respiratory infections

▲ cerebellar degeneration

▲ poly-substance abuse (time of last use?)

3. Signs of alcohol intoxication:

▲ unsteady gait

▲ incoordination

▲ nystagmus

▲ belligerence

▲ impaired attention

▲ loss of inhibition

▲ memory loss

▲ hypertension

▲ coma

▲ odor of alcohol

▲ mood lability

▲ impaired judgment

▲ vomiting

▲ palpitations

▲ stupor

▲ slurred speech

▲ confusion

▲ cardiac arrhythmias

▲ altered level of perception

4. Signs of alcohol withdrawal:

May *begin* 6 to 8 hours after cessation or reduction of the alcohol intake, and symptoms will *peak* in approximately 24 to 48 hours. (For facts about withdrawal and delirium tremens, see Box 2–6).

▲ Stage 1

• anxiety

• tachycardia

• nausea/vomiting

• headache

• insomnia

• dehydration

• tremors

• diaphoresis

■ Box 2–6: FACTS ABOUT WITHDRAWAL AND DELERIUM TREMENS

• Mortality rate for delerium tremens (DT) is 20%.

• DTs are preventable with sedatives.

• It is difficult to predict which patients will develop a major withdrawal reaction; therefore, it is reasonable to sedate all patients who are recently abstinent from alcohol.

• It is difficult to control a severe withdrawal reaction once it begins; therefore, aggressive therapy of all early abstinence patients is important.

• Large doses of sedatives may be required to prevent severe withdrawal reaction and DTs.

- nightmares
- anorexia
- hypertension
- hypovolemia
- irritability
- depression
- jerky muscle movements
- hyperthermia
- positive orthostatic vital signs
▲ Stage 2
- hallucinations (tactile, visual, auditory)
- intensification of stage 1 symptoms
▲ Stage 3
- paranoia
- delirium
- disorientation
- delusions
- amnesia
- intensification of stage 1 and 2 symptoms
▲ Stage 4
- seizures

 ALERT   Appropriate identification and treatment *before* the development of stages 1 and 2 **prevent** stages 3 and 4.

B. If suspicion of alcoholism exists, perform a more specific substance abuse assessment.
1. History of substances:
   ▲ age substance first used
   ▲ frequency, amount, and duration of use
   ▲ date or time of last use for each of the following:
   - alcohol
   - cocaine/crack
   - cannabis
   - depressants
   - heroin
   - inhalants
   - hallucinogens
   - stimulants
   - other (including prescribed medications)
2. History of:
   ▲ withdrawal
   ▲ tolerance

    ▲ previous treatment programs (including when and where)
- inpatient
- outpatient
- self-help
- success with previous programs
- family history of substance abuse

3. **CAGE** questions:
    ▲ **C** Have you ever attempted to *cut down* on your use?
    ▲ **A** Have you ever been *annoyed* when others mention your use?
    ▲ **G** Have you ever felt *guilty* about your use?
    ▲ **E** Have you ever needed an *"eye opener"*?

! ALERT   Two or three "yes" answers to these questions strongly suggest chemical dependence.

! ALERT   Withdrawal from alcohol is a potentially lethal process.

Interventions

1. Complete primary and secondary survey with interventions as indicated.
2. Assess for suicidal behavior.
3. Check blood pressure, pulse, and temperature readings hourly for the first 8 to 12 hours after admission.
    ▲ Vital signs should be assessed at least every 4 hours for the first 48 hours after admission (Varcarolis, 1998).
    ▲ The pulse is a good indicator of progression into and through withdrawal.
    ▲ Elevated pulse may indicate pending alcohol withdrawal delirium.
4. Obtain IV access for rehydration.
    ▲ Because of hypoglycemia, hypokalemia, hypomagnesemia, and thiamine deficiency that are common to the alcoholic person, replacements must be given at the time of IV initiation.

! ALERT   Thiamine must be replaced before the administration of glucose to prevent the development of Wernicke-Korsakoff syndrome.

---

5. Administer medication as patient progresses through withdrawal. (Phenobarbital and lorazepam are most commonly used.)

Alzheimer's Disease

- ▲ A disease of the brain that causes a steady decline in memory and intellectual functioning
- ▲ An estimated 4 million Americans have Alzheimer's disease
- ▲ Third leading cause of death in the elderly
- ▲ An estimated 10% of people over age 65 have Alzheimer's disease
- ▲ An estimated 30% to 50% of those over 85 have Alzheimer's disease

Assessment

A. Perform a general mental health assessment per protocol.
  1. Associated information:
     - ▲ complete medical history and triage assessment
     - ▲ may need to interview family members for a complete assessment of the patient's current status
  2. Associated signs and symptoms:
     - ▲ Subtle changes in memory, often reported by family members first and include:
       - • forgetfulness
       - • repetitiveness
       - • difficulty organizing thoughts
       - • social withdrawal
       - • difficulty processing information
     - ▲ See Table 2–17 for differences between age-appropriate memory loss and Alzheimer's disease.
     - ▲ As the disease progresses, additional issues arise:
       - • language skills diminish
       - • decreased ability to perform calculations or plan activities
       - • difficulty in performing personal hygiene or daily activities such as showering, dressing, shopping
     - ▲ Aphasia
       - • initially, the person has a hard time finding the right word to use
       - • over time, the person's vocabulary diminishes greatly, until he or she is finally reduced to babbling or becoming mute

TABLE 2–17 • Memory/Loss Comparison: Normal Aging Versus Alzheimer's Disease

Activity	Age-Appropriate Memory Loss	Alzheimer's Disease
Forgets an experience	May forget parts of an experience	Forgets the whole experience
Remembers the experience later	Often	Rarely
Can follow written or spoken directions	Usually able to follow directions	Gradually unable to follow any directions
Can keep notes to help one's memory	Usually able to do this and finds it very helpful	Gradually unable to use notes to help with memory
Able to provide care for self	Usually able to provide most of own care	Gradually unable to care for self

▲ Apraxia
  • the person loses purposeful movement in the absence of motor or sensory impairment
  • forgets how to dress, put on shoes, walk, etc.
▲ Agnosia
  • lose the ability to recognize objects, sounds, and people that were once familiar
▲ Mnemonic disturbance
  • person starts with memory loss of recent events and gradually progresses to include both recent and remote events.

 Interventions:

1. Always identify yourself and call the patient by his or her name during EVERY interaction.
2. Speak slowly, using short, simple phrases.
3. Maintain face-to-face contact.
4. Talk about things that are familiar to the patient.
5. Reinforce reality–avoid arguing or refuting delusions.
6. Have patient perform all tasks he or she is capable of.
7. Allow patient to wear own clothes whenever possible.
8. Minimize sensory stimulation.

 ALERT   Health care providers must always facilitate the highest level of functioning for all cognitively impaired patients.

▶ *Bipolar Disorder (Manic/Depression)*

▲ Bipolar disorder is a mood disorder characterized by alternating manic and depressive episodes.
▲ Manic episodes include extremely labile excitement, hyperactivity, and euphoria.
▲ Depressive episodes include extreme sadness, slowed thought process, and marked fatigue.
▲ The patient may have long periods of normal and stable moods between elevated and depressed moods.

ALERT   Patient is a **threat** to self and others until *mania* is controlled or severe *depression* is relieved.

Assessment

A. Perform a general mental health assessment per protocol.
  1. Associated information:
     ▲ complete medical history and triage assessment
     ▲ organic causes of depression
     ▲ electroconvulsive therapy that may precipitate a manic episode
     ▲ medication that may cause episodes of mania:
       • antidepressants
       • amphetamines
       • steroids
     ▲ medications that may cause depression:
       • antihypertensives
       • oral contraceptives
       • steroids
       • narcotics
       • antiparkinsonian drugs
       • amphetamines
       • barbiturates
     ▲ family history of bipolar illness
     ▲ previous episodes of manic/depression
  2. Associated signs and symptoms of mania:
     ▲ three most common symptoms of mania include:
       • elated mood
       • increased activity
       • reduced sleep
     ▲ other signs and symptoms include:
       • flight of ideas
       • grandiosity
       • inflated self-esteem
       • impaired mentation
       • flamboyant actions
       • disorganized behavior
       • hyperactivity
       • auditory hallucinations
       • psychosis
       • increased sexual energy
       • impairment of rational thought
       • poor social judgment
       • hostile or paranoid behavior when stressed
       • impulsive behavior
       • sleep impairment
       • rapid or pressured speech
       • excessive spending
       • boundless enthusiasm
  3. Associated signs and symptoms of depression (see Mental Health/Depression).

Interventions

1. Complete primary and secondary survey with interventions as indicated.
2. Provide for patient safety.
   ▲ Security officers
   ▲ Possibility of chemical and/or physical restraints
3. Remain emotionally separated from patient's behavior.
   ▲ Although the patient may present as humorous, joking, and full of energy, the nurse must remain professional at all times, utilizing BRIEF interactions with the patient.
   ▲ Move the patient from a stimulating environment into a quiet one.
   ▲ Set limits and enforce them.
      • the manic patient may attempt to control decisions and boundaries
      • staff must follow established policies and plans of care for this patient

Borderline Personality Disorder

▲ These patients are borderline between psychosis and neurosis.
▲ Patients are plagued by problems of identity and unstable interpersonal relationships.

Assessment

A. Perform a general mental health assessment per protocol.
   1. Associated signs, symptoms, and characteristics:
      ▲ unstable interpersonal relationships
      ▲ poor self image
      ▲ fear of abandonment and/or rejection–clinging, lonely behavior
      ▲ impulsive behavior
      ▲ sexual promiscuity
      ▲ suicidal ideation
      ▲ inappropriate overreaction to stress
      ▲ constant criticism of others
      ▲ self-mutilating behavior (especially cutting)
      ▲ rapid, intense mood swings
      ▲ frequently expresses anger towards those that are trying to help them or those that are close to them
      ▲ difficult, hostile, emotional, and demanding behaviors, often provokes anger and rejection response from caretakers
      ▲ splitting and manipulative behaviors—very good at pitting one person against another with their behavior and comments
   2. Past history often includes:
      ▲ depression
      ▲ chronic feelings of emptiness
      ▲ substance abuse
      ▲ physical and/or sexual abuse as a child

> **! ALERT** Patients with a borderline personality are a major risk for suicide. They can be manipulative and cunning—treat them as suicidal until **PROVEN** otherwise.

 Interventions

1. Decrease the number of staff involved in the care of this patient.
   ▲ Must maintain consistency among staff when working with this patient
2. Use structured, clear, brief interactions.
3. Explain behavioral expectations to patient.
4. Avoid focusing on negative behavior.
5. Establish limits, especially on the nursing time spent with patient.
6. Point out to patient when he or she attempts to be manipulative and how these behaviors are counterproductive.
7. Reinforce the patient's "**behavior** is unacceptable," but avoid implying that the patient is unacceptable.

▶ *Depression*

- ▲ Depression is an affective disorder that affects most people at some point in their life.
- ▲ It causes intense emotional pain and suffering.
- ▲ Depression potentially may be linked to suicide.
- ▲ It can be difficult to diagnose since it is easily masked by somatic symptoms and has a variety of manifestations, intensities, and etiologies.
- ▲ Depression affects at least 10 million Americans.
- ▲ It is difficult to diagnose in adolescence because:
  - teens may be ambivalent about sharing feelings with adults
  - symptoms may be dismissed as "a stage they're going through"
  - acting-out behavior may mask depression

Assessment

A. Perform a general mental health assessment per protocol.
   1. Associated information:
      ▲ complete medical history and triage assessment
      ▲ rule out:
         - possibility of organic cause of depression
         - increased use of alcohol, prescriptions, or OTC medications
         - use of medications or illicit drugs that may cause depression (Table 2–18):
            – antihypertensives
            – oral contraceptives
            – steroids
            – narcotics

TABLE 2–18 • Drugs of Abuse

Drug Name/Type	Street Name	Method Used	Physical Effects	Mental Effects
ALCOHOL CNS depressant	Booze Hooch Juice Brew	Swallowed in liquid form	Blurs vision, slurs speech, alters coordination, heart and liver damage, addiction, gastric and esophageal ulcers, brain damage, blackouts, hypoglycemia, anemia, Wernicke-Korsakoff syndrome, oral cancer, fetal alcohol syndrome, death from overdose	Scrambles thought process, impairs judgement, memory loss, alters perception, delirium, apathy
COCAINE CNS stimulant	Coke C-dust Snow Toot White lady Blow Rock(s) Crack Flake Big "C" Happy dust Bernice Horse Fluff Caine Coconut Icing Mojo Zip	Smoked/free basing, inhaled/ snorted, injected, swallowed in powder, pill, or rock form	Rapidly metabolized, producing a brief high of <30 minutes Chronic use can result in cocaine psychosis, a condition similar to paranoid schizophrenia Intense psychological dependence Dilated pupils, profuse sweating, runny nose, dry mouth, tachycardia, hypertension, insomnia, anorexia, indifference to pain, destruction of nasal septum, heart and lung damage, death from overdose	Euphoria, illusive mental or physical power, extreme mood swings, restlessness, hallucinations, paranoia, psychosis, severe depression, anxiety, formication
CNS DEPRESSANTS Barbiturates phenobarbital: Luminal amobarbital: Amytal secobarbital: Seconal pentobarbital: Nembutal sodium pentothal	Reds Barbs Yellow jackets Red devils Blue devils Yellow submarine Blues and reds Idiot pills Sleepers Stumblers Downers	IV injection, suppository, swallowed in pill form	Drowsiness, slurred speech, skeletal muscle relaxation, poor muscle control, incoordination, nausea, slowed reaction time, involuntary eye movements, hypotension, bradycardia, bradypnea, constricted pupils, clammy skin, loss of appetite Penetrates the placental wall, addiction is passed to the baby	Confusion, impaired judgment, impaired performance, anxiety and tension followed by a sense of calm, mood swings, forgetfulness

TABLE 2–18 • Drugs of Abuse (Continued)

Drug Name/Type	Street Name	Method Used	Physical Effects	Mental Effects
CNS DEPRESSANTS (continued)			Withdrawal is prolonged and severe—symptoms range from temporary psychosis to cardiac arrest Cellulitis at injection site Chronic use results in extreme psychological and physical addiction; death from overdose	
Nonbarbiturates Methaqualone Quaalude Soper	Downers Ludes Soapers Wallbangers Lemons Lovers Quack 714s 300s	Swallowed in pill form	Same as barbiturates Physically and psychologically addictive Withdrawal is *very* difficult Severe interaction with alcohol Death from overdose	Same as barbiturates
Tranquilizers, Benzodiazepines (Reduces tension and anxiety without sedating)				
diazepam: Valium chlordiazepoxide: Libruim lorazepam: Ativan oxazepam: Serax alprazolam: Xanax	Downers	Injection, swallowed in pill form	Decreased reflex action, vision changes, muscle relaxation, hypotension, bradycardia, slurred speech, drowsiness, blurred vision; prolonged use causes severe physical and psychological addiction	Alteration in spatial judgment and sense of time, sense of calm, impaired judgment, confusion, depression, hallucinations
HALLUCINOGENS (Drugs that alter perceptions of reality)				
PCP	Angel dust Killer Black whack Supergrass Peace pill Sherms Superweed DOA CJ Goon dust Dust joint Live one Mad dog T-buzz Wobble Weed Zombie	Swallowed in pill form, sprayed on a cigarette and smoked	Drooling, nystagmus, restlessness, incoordination, rigid muscles, tachycardia, hypertension, superhuman strength, dulled sensations to touch and pain, impaired speech Death is common, but from accidents, not from overdose Extremely dangerous drug since it is a narcotic, stimulant, depressant, and hallucinogen A "trip" is a cycle of stimulation, depression, hallucination, which then repeats itself, lasting 2–14 hours	Disorientation, amnesia, anxiety, depression, confusion, agitation, violent, hostile, suicidal, extreme personality changes

TABLE 2–18 • Drugs of Abuse (Continued)

Drug Name/Type	Street Name	Method Used	Physical Effects	Mental Effects
LSD	Acid Blue heaven Instant Zen Purple hearts Pure love Sugar cubes Tail lights	Swallowed in liquid form, dropped on sugar cube, sprayed on paper tablet	Nausea, tachycardia, tachypnea, hyperthermia, hypertension, dilated pupils, diaphoresis, palpitations, incoordination; trips last 4–14 hours; heightens all 5 senses	Altered reality perception, psychotic disturbances, paranoia, synesthesia, hallucinations, mood swings, terrifying flashbacks
Mescaline Psilocybin	Mesc Moon Peyote Buttons	Swallowed in natural form	Same as LSD	Same as LSD
INHALANTS				
Gasoline Airplane glue Paint thinner Drycleaner fluid Nitrous oxide		Inhaled or sniffed using a paper or plastic bag or rag	Incoordination, impaired vision, neuropathy, muscle weakness, anemia, vertigo, headache, weight loss,	Memory and thought impairment, depression, aggression, hostility, paranoia, abusive
	Laughing gas Whippets Buzz bomb Nitro	Inhaled or sniffed by mask or balloons	nausea, vomiting, sneezing, coughing, nosebleeds, slurred speech, tachycardia, fatigue,	behavior, mood swings, withdrawal from family and friends, violent behavior
Amyl nitrite Butyl nitrite	Poppers Snappers Pearls Aimies Bolt Climax Thrust	Inhaled or sniffed from gauze or ampules	dilated pupils, chemical smell on breath, brain, liver, and bone marrow damage, death by anoxia	
MARIJUANA/HASHISH (CNS depressant)				
	Joint Grass Hash Pot "J" Maryjane Reefer Colombian Locoweed Love weed	Smoked, swallowed in solid form	Interferes with psychological maturation, psychological dependence	Sensory distortion, decrease in motivation, forgetfulness, confusion, anxiety, paranoia
NARCOTICS (Natural or synthetic drug that contains or resembles opium; CNS depressants)				
Dilaudid	Dillys Cowboys	Swallowed in pill or liquid form, injected	Drowsiness, lethargy, hypotension, bradycardia, muscle weakness, death from overdose	Forgetfulness, sedation, sense of peace
Percodan	Perks Pink spoons			
Demerol Methadone	Peth Dollies			

TABLE 2–18 • Drugs of Abuse (Continued)

Drug Name/Type	Street Name	Method Used	Physical Effects	Mental Effects
NARCOTICS (Natural or synthetic drug that contains or resembles opium; CNS depressants) *(continued)*				
	Amidone			
	Fizzies			
Codeine	Schoolboy	Swallowed in		
	Cody	pill or liquid		
	Threes	form		
	Fours			
Morphine	Mojo	Smoked,	Tolerance occurs quickly,	Produces an intense
	Morphy	IV injection	addiction occurs in as	orgasmic rush followed by
	Mud		little as 1–3 weeks	euphoria, peace, and a
	Dreamer		Withdrawal is painful,	comforting warmth;
	Miss Emma		with intense cramps, cold	confusion, forgetfulness,
			sweats, delirium, pain,	stupor
			fever, headaches, and	
			seizures lasting ~ 4 days	
Heroin	Horse			
	Junk			
	Dope			
	Blanco			
	Black pearl			
	Bonita			
STIMULANTS (Cause CNS stimulation)				
Amphetamines	Hi speed	Pill form,	Body enters a state of stress	Extreme exhilaration and
Benzadrine	Lip poppers	injected,	Anorexia, tachycardia,	stimulation, inflated
Biphetamine	Speckled	snorted	palpitations, hypertension,	confidence, irritability,
	birds		inability to sleep, nasal and	volatile, aggressive,
Dextroamphetamine	Dexies		bronchial passages enlarge,	nervousness, mood
Dexedrine	Brownies		restriction of cerebral	swings, hallucinations,
Synatan	Brown and		blood flow, dilated pupils,	paranoia, formication,
Appetral	clears		sweating, restlessness,	psychosis, hypomania
Methamphetamine	Speed		muscle tremors, rapid and	
Methedrine	Meth		garbled speech, excessive	
Desoxyn	Crystal		activity, brain damage,	
Ambar	Crank		seizures, CVA, coma, death	
	Crypto		from overdose	
	Ice		Drug effects last 4–14 hours	
	Yellow bam		"Speeding" occurs with	
			injection, causing user to	
			go ~5 days without sleep	
			Causes birth defects	
			Extreme physical and	
			psychological addiction	
Herbal Stimulants				
Ephedrine	Ultimate	Pill, powder,	Same as above	Extreme exhilaration and
	Xphoria	liquid	Often marketed as safe	stimulation, inflated
	Herbal ecstasy		and legal alternatives	confidence, reduced

TABLE 2–18 • Drugs of Abuse (Continued)

Drug Name/Type	Street Name	Method Used	Physical Effects	Mental Effects
STIMULANTS (Cause CNS stimulation) *(continued)*				
	Legal weed		to street drugs	inhibitions, euphoria,
	Buzz tablets		Heightened sexual sensation,	happy and friendly,
	Cloud 9		higher energy level,	empathy towards others,
	Black		tachycardia, sweating,	irritability, volatile,
	Lemonade		body tremors, dilated	aggressive, nervousness,
	Brainalizer		pupils, muscle spasms,	mood swings,
	Fungalore		grinding of teeth,	hallucinations, paranoia,
	Herbal XTC		elevated blood pressure	formication, psychosis,
	Planet X		Easily obtainable on the	hypomania
	The Drink		Internet, through magazines,	
	X Tablets		and at stores such as	
	Brain wash		convenience markets,	
	Buzz tablets		health food stores, and	
	Fukola cola		"head shops"	
	Love potion #69			
	Naturally high			
	Rave energy			
	Love drug			
	Adam			
	XTC			
	X			
ANESTHETICS				
GHB and Analogs	Liquid X	Oral	Onset is 10–20 minutes	Mood swings, amnesia,
	Liquid		Duration is 2–3 hours	sleepy, drunken
	Ecstasy		Slow slurred speech, loss	appearance
	Water		of muscle coordination,	
	"G"		nausea, vomiting,	
	Easy lay		bradycardia or tachycardia,	
			hypotension, hypothermic	
			Overdose: cardiac and	
			respiratory arrest, seizures,	
			incontinences of stool and	
			urine, unconsciousness	
Ketamine	K	Injected, snorted,	Onset is immediate if smoked	Euphoria, paranoia, anxiety,
	Super K	smoked, oral,	or injected	disorientation, violence,
	Special K	rectal	Duration is 1–2 hours	agitation, insomnia,
	God		About 1/4 the strength of	delusions, pain relief,
	Jet		PCP, depending on the dose	intoxication,
	Honey oil		used	hallucinations, sleepy
	Blast		Sweating, slurred or slow	appearance, confusion
	Gas		speech, muscle rigidity, blank	
			stare, elevated body	
			temperature, tachycardia,	
			loss of muscle coordination,	
			hypertension, excess strength	

- antiparkinsonian drugs
- amphetamines
- barbiturates
- inhalants
• situational crisis
• loss of significant other
• sudden health changes
• separation from spiritual source or normal support system
• childbirth
• change in occupational status

2. Associated signs and symptoms:
   ▲ extreme fatigue
   ▲ anhedonia
   ▲ changes in appetite
   ▲ overwhelming sense of hopelessness and helplessness
   ▲ persistent irritability
   ▲ sense of guilt or worthlessness
   ▲ somatic complaints with no organic cause
   ▲ forgetfulness
   ▲ impairment of sleep pattern
      • difficulty falling asleep
      • difficulty staying asleep
      • excessive sleep
   ▲ psychomotor agitation
      • depressed mood
      • crying
   ▲ psychomotor retardation
      • slowed metabolism
      • monotone voice
      • constipation
      • slowed speech process
      • minimal body movement
      • slowed thought process
   ▲ thoughts of death or suicide

 ALERT   Thoughts of suicide should **ALWAYS** be taken seriously. Complete a suicide risk assessment.

---

3. Age-related considerations:
   ▲ pediatric patients may present with:
      • hyperactivity
      • enuresis

- regression
- aggression
- sadness
- sleeping problems
- irritability
- anxiety
- suicidal ideation
- misbehavior
- restlessness
- change in appetite

▲ adolescents may present with:
  - acting-out behaviors
  - delinquency
  - detached from others
  - anger or hostility
  - hopelessness
  - alcohol and drug abuse
  - aggression
  - suicidal ideation
  - verbal sarcasm
  - traumatic injuries
  - school issues
  - disillusionment
  - loneliness
  - sexual promiscuity
  - overeating or anorexia
  - conduct disorders
  - running away from home
  - preoccupation with death

! ALERT Persistent or sudden signs of change can be key in identification of depression in adolescence.

▲ elderly may present with:
  - apathy
  - loss of appetite
  - insomnia
  - weight loss
  - mood swings
  - easy agitation
  - pessimism
  - extreme fatigue

- low self-esteem
- suicidal thoughts
- profound memory impairment
- very unsociable behavior
- change in sleep patterns
- decreased sexual activity
- heightened concerns for bodily functions
- increased anxiety and fear for no reason
- feelings of insignificance
- inability to concentrate
- poor personal hygiene
- delusions of persecution or somatic theme

 ALERT A depressed elderly person may appear to have dementia, not depression. Assess *carefully!*

 Interventions

1. Complete primary and secondary survey with interventions, as indicated.
2. Assess for patient safety and assign patient to treatment area, as necessary.
3. Arrange for 1:1 observation if patient is at risk for suicide.
4. Form a therapeutic relationship with the patient that includes excellent communication skills, empathy, acceptance, trust, and compassion.
5. Avoid labeling an elderly patient as having dementia until a complete mental health assessment has been performed.
6. If you suspect that a depressed patient may be suicidal, ask:
   - ▲ "Sometimes when people feel this depressed/hopeless/sad, they have thoughts of hurting or killing themselves. Have you ever had thoughts like these?"
   - ▲ If the patient answers "yes," then assess the following:
     - Does the person have a plan?
     - Assess lethality of plan (handful of aspirin versus a gun).
     - Does person have the means to carry out the plan?
     - Does he or she have access to a gun, poison, car, etc.?
     - Has person ever attempted suicide before?

▶ *Eating Disorders*

- ▲ 50 million Americans are on a weight-loss regimen.
- ▲ A small portion of those suffer from a true psychiatric eating disorder.
- ▲ Two primary eating disorders are anorexia nervosa and bulimia.
- ▲ Obesity is sometimes considered the third eating disorder.

Anorexia Nervosa

▲ Deep-seated roots of this disorder are emotional and psychological.
▲ Cause of anorexia is unknown, although often will include:
  • someone of normal weight who begins to diet and eventually begins suppressing hunger sensations to the point of self-starvation
  • a history of someone in the family who is a dieter, overweight, or focused on staying slim and fit
▲ Classic patients lose 15% to 35% of their original body weight.

Assessment

A. Perform a general mental health assessment per protocol.
  1. Signs and symptoms:
     ▲ large weight loss in short period of time
     ▲ continues to diet although bone thin
     ▲ reaches diet goal and immediately sets another goal for further weight loss
     ▲ remains dissatisfied with appearance, claiming to feel fat even after reaching weight-loss goal
     ▲ prefers dieting in isolation (instead of joining a group)
     ▲ amenorrhea
     ▲ has an unusual interest in food
     ▲ strange eating rituals such as cutting food into tiny pieces or measuring all food before consumption
     ▲ becomes a "closet" eater
     ▲ obsessive about exercising
     ▲ depressed
     ▲ may begin to binge and purge

Interventions

1. Patient needs a multidisciplinary plan of care.
2. Immediate care in the ED includes treating immediate health issues.
3. Refer patient to psychological treatment service.

Bulimia

▲ Deep-seated roots of this disorder are emotional and psychological.
▲ Bulimia usually begins with a diet that leads to binging and purging.
▲ Highest risk between the ages of 17 to 25 years old, although a delay in diagnosis may occur until the patient is in the 30s or 40s.

Assessment

A. Perform a general mental healthy assessment per protocol.
  1. Signs and symptoms:
     ▲ may be slightly underweight or overweight

▲ irregular menstrual cycle

▲ diminished sexual interest

▲ impulsive behaviors:
  • shoplifting
  • alcohol and drug abuse

▲ may appear healthy, successful—often perfectionists

▲ very low self-esteem

▲ eats in secret

▲ eats enormous amounts of food but does not gain weight

▲ goes to the bathroom for an extended period of time after meals (to induce vomiting)

▲ depression

▲ scars on the back of hands from forced vomiting

▲ purging
  • use of laxatives
  • use of diuretics
  • self-induced vomiting

▲ excessive exercising

▲ binges regularly, then purges

▲ binge—purge cycle causes:
  • electrolyte imbalance
    – sodium
    – magnesium
    – potassium
    – calcium

▲ fatigue

▲ seizures

▲ muscle cramps

▲ irregular heartbeat

▲ decreased bone density

▲ esophageal damage

▲ receding gum line

▲ eroded tooth enamel

▲ rash

▲ broken blood vessels in the cheeks

▲ swelling
  • around the eyes
  • ankles
  • feet
  • neck glands

Interventions

1. Patient needs a multidisciplinary plan of care.
2. Immediate care in the ED includes treating immediate health issues.
3. Refer patient to psychological treatment service.

Obesity

- ▲ 97 million American adults are overweight.
- ▲ Obesity is measured using the body mass index (BMI).
- ▲ This is determined by dividing the person's weight in kilograms by a person's height in meters squared.
  - Overweight: BMI of 25–29.9 kg/m^2
  - Obesity: 30–39.9 kg/m^2
  - Extreme obesity: >40 kg/m^2
- ▲ Obesity is a complex condition caused by a variety of factors:
  - behavioral
  - cultural
  - genetic
  - metabolic
  - physiologic
  - social

Assessment

A. Perform a general health assessment per protocol.
  1. Assess comorbidities
     - ▲ If a patient has any of these, they are considered to be at a high absolute risk for death. *These problems need immediate treatment*:
       - atherosclerosis
       - peripheral artery disease
       - carotid artery disease
       - coronary artery disease
       - myocardial infarction
       - cardiac bypass surgery
       - sleep apnea
       - type 2 diabetes
     - ▲ dangerous but not life-threatening risks:
       - gallstones
       - gynecologic problems (amenorrhea)
       - osteoarthritis
       - stress incontinence
     - ▲ If three of these comorbidities are combined, there is an increased risk of death:
       - men >45 years of age
       - women >55 years of age
       - cigarette smoker
       - family history of early heart disease
       - hypertension
       - high-LDL cholesterol
       - impaired fasting glucose levels
       - low-HDL cholesterol

2. Long-term effects of obesity:
   ▲ back pain
   ▲ breathing problems
   ▲ certain types of cancer
   ▲ coronary heart disease
   ▲ diabetes
   ▲ gallbladder disease
   ▲ hypertension
   ▲ osteoarthritis
   ▲ stroke

Interventions

1. Airway management and breathing:
   ▲ May need two people to use the bag-valve-mask.
   ▲ Intubation may be difficult —be prepared for difficulties.
   ▲ Patient may need to be in "sitting" position to aid intubation procedure.
   ▲ Auscultation of breath sounds will be distant.
   ▲ Percutaneous cricothyrotomy or surgical tracheostomy may be difficult.
   ▲ Obstructive sleep apnea is common.
2. Nursing care:
   ▲ Use a large (thigh) cuff for blood pressures; may need to use the distal portion of the arm.
   ▲ Be sure to use the help of others when moving or positioning the patient.
   ▲ Use appropriately sized equipment for the patient:
     • wheelchairs
     • cane, crutches, walker
     • bedside commode
   ▲ Good skin care is essential to prevent bed sores and cellulitis.
   ▲ Foley catheters
     • male patients may need to have suprapubic skin folds and adipose tissue retracted with the heel of the provider's hand or the assist of another before the catheter is inserted.
     • female patients will need the assistance of another provider to hold skin folds clear of the insertion site during the procedure
   ▲ Use a blood pressure cuff instead of a tourniquet when drawing blood samples or placing an IV.
   ▲ May need to select a longer needle when giving injections.
   ▲ May need to use extra-long needles during a lumbar puncture (5.5 inch).
3. Personal care:
   ▲ If you are uncertain as how to best adapt care to the patient, consider asking the patient:
     • "How do you do this at home?"
     • "How would you like us to help?"
   ▲ A typical ED stretcher may not be safe for an obese patient. Consider obtaining a regular bed for the patient.
   ▲ May be difficult for the patient who can't see or reach the part of his or her body that needs cleaning
   ▲ Rashes and chafing may be common inside of skin folds that occur (yeast and fungus are common).

▶ *Explosive and Inflexible Youth*

▲ Our young patients may present for any number of conditions or concerns and have an underlying history of being explosive or inflexible.

▲ These children can pose a great challenge to the triage nurse, trying to work efficiently—and to the ED nurse who tries to render appropriate care to this child.

▲ Understanding these children will help the ED experience be a successful one for the child, the caretaker, and for the ED staff.

▲ Characteristics of children who are explosive and inflexible:
  • they do not possess the skills to tolerate rising frustration levels
  • in general, they do not respond to traditional motivational approaches
  • symptoms are often thought to occur from neurologic impairment as opposed to psychological reasons
  • prone to stubborn, inflexible, explosive outbursts

▲ When dealing with these children, the ED nurse should:
  • avoid labeling the child by his or her challenges
  • avoid prejudging the child
  • control his or her own frustration and anger
    – don't take the child's behavior personally
    – don't allow the child's behavior to stimulate a rise in your own anger and frustration
  • remember that when a child threatens us ("I'm going to run away"), that's really a request to know how much you care about him or her
    – avoid telling the child to "go ahead"—instead, say "It's been a long day for you and it would be sad if you ran away."
    – inflexible and explosive children challenge the adults in their world to determine whether they are truly cared about or not.
  • understand that these children try to push others away from them as a way of protecting themselves
    – if a child has behavior that is irritating and unacceptable, the health care provider should respond with "It feels like you're trying to push me away. I'd like to help you feel better—will you let me help?"
  • caregivers should speak softly and *respond* to the child's behavior. *Avoid* reacting—*always* keep your cool.
  • to manage teenagers successfully, we need to first successfully manage ourselves.
  • find something that makes the child feel successful and focus on that throughout the ED visit. You'll find the child more willing to work with you instead of work against you.
  • kids in need can't deal with bad moods of their health care providers.
    – they tend to believe they again failed in life by doing something that made the health care worker displeased with the child.
  • explosive and inflexible children need to know the rules to succeed.
    – communicate with the children, share with them the expectations while in the ED, and the expected course. Keep them updated frequently.
  • **Use distraction to diffuse an angry child BEFORE he or she explodes.**

Obsessive/Compulsive Disorder (OCD)

▲ An *obsession* is a persistent, intrusive, or unwanted thought or image that cannot be eliminated by reason or logic.

▲ *Compulsions* are repetitive behaviors performed to reduce or to prevent the intense anxiety associated with the obsessive thought.

▲ Mild obsessive/compulsive symptoms are similar to someone who "worries too much." These obsessions are often socially acceptable (e.g., being on time) and only mildly annoying.

▲ More serious obsessive/compulsive behaviors involve sexuality, violence, germs, illness, or death. Those with a profound obsessive/compulsive disorder experience interpersonal, social, and economic dysfunction.

▲ Depression is commonly suffered by patients with OCD.

Assessment

A. Perform a general mental health assessment per protocol.
   1. Associated information:
      ▲ may be ultimate perfectionist
      ▲ great fear of making a mistake or being wrong
      ▲ high emotional need to be in control
   2. Associated signs and symptoms:
      ▲ skin or dental trauma from repeated cleansing
      ▲ lack of appropriate coping skills
      ▲ moderate to severe anxiety
      ▲ impaired interpersonal relationships
      ▲ fear
      ▲ hypochondriacal behavior
      ▲ pathological sense of guilt
      ▲ chemical dependency
   3. Common obsessive thoughts:
      ▲ checking and double-checking
      ▲ sexual imagery or ideation
      ▲ violent thought or acts against self or others
      ▲ intense fear of germs or dirt
      ▲ fear of illness or death
   4. Common compulsive behaviors:
      ▲ counting (stairs, doors, cups, etc.)
      ▲ touching (doorknobs, religious objects, etc.)
      ▲ washing (hands, surfaces, objects, etc.)
      ▲ avoiding (touching, people, groups, etc.)
      ▲ doing/undoing (gets up from a chair and sits down again repeatedly)
      ▲ symmetry (placing objects in perfect alignment, mandatory sequence, etc.)

Interventions

1. Complete primary and secondary survey with intervention, as indicated.
2. Assess for patient safety and assign patient to treatment area, as necessary.
3. Allow the patient time to complete the compulsive tasks.
4. Develop rapport with the patient to help decrease his or her heightened anxiety level.
5. Emphasize the patient's strengths.

▶ *Panic Attack/Disorder*

▲ A spontaneous yet terrorizing emotional event experienced by a patient
▲ This emotionally paralyzing event lasts for 3 to 10 minutes and may include:
- suspension of normal function
- dramatically narrowed perceptual field
- misinterpretation of reality
- overwhelming fear or dread
- physical symptoms such as chest pain, shortness of breath, etc.

▲ Many patients experiencing panic attacks may also suffer with depression.

Assessment

A. Perform a general mental health assessment per protocol.
1. Associated information:
   ▲ complete medical history and triage assessment
   ▲ situation that may precipitate a panic attack:
   - hypoglycemia
   - caffeine use
   - withdrawal from alcohol or tranquilizers
   - stressful event
   - sudden loss or life change
2. Associated signs and symptoms:
   ▲ tachycardia
   ▲ dyspnea
   ▲ chest pain
   ▲ dizziness
   ▲ numbness, hands or feet
   ▲ delusions
   ▲ tremors
   ▲ overwhelming fear of losing control, going crazy, or dying
   ▲ palpitations
   ▲ tachypnea
   ▲ cool, clammy skin

▲ syncope
▲ hot or cold flashes
▲ hallucinations
▲ loss of reality orientation

 Interventions

1. Complete primary and secondary survey with interventions, as indicated.
2. Rule out physical cause for symptoms.
3. Provide for patient safety.
4. Stay with patient while offering reassurance.
5. Remove patient from stimulating environment.

Schizophrenia

▲ A pathologic process resulting in psychotic behavior (acute or chronic)
▲ A severe disturbance in thought process, affect, behavior, and perception
▲ Impairment of reality orientation
▲ Severe withdrawal from reality and seclusion into a private world of his or her own
▲ Symptoms usually manifest during adolescence or early adulthood
▲ Slow onset, from 1 month to 2 years before the first psychotic break; may see gradual deterioration from previous level of functioning

 Assessment

A. Perform a general mental health assessment per protocol.
  1. Associated information:
    ▲ complete medical history and triage assessment
    ▲ affect:
      • blunted
      • inappropriate
      • flat
      • bizarre
    ▲ behavioral effects:
      • acting-out behavior
      • impulsiveness
      • catatonia
      • psychomotor retardation
      • psychomotor agitation
      • bizarre behaviors (e.g., eccentric dress)
    ▲ perceptual effects:
      • illusions
      • derealization

- hallucinations
- autism
- depersonalization
- thinking not bound to reality

▲ impaired thought process:
- delusions
- incoherence
- paranoia
- neologisms
- looseness of association
- confused
- illogical thought
- illogical speech (i.e., word salad)

▲ functional psychosis includes:
- schizophrenia
- mania
- psychotic depression
- brief reactive psychosis

▲ organic psychoses includes:
- dementia
- delirium
- toxic drug psychosis

2. Associated signs and symptoms:
   ▲ anhedonia
   ▲ acute or chronic anxiety
   ▲ loss of concentration
   ▲ loneliness
   ▲ lack of self-respect
   ▲ feelings of rejection
   ▲ compulsions and/or obsessions
   ▲ apathy
   ▲ uncommunicative speech
   ▲ delusions and/or hallucinations
   ▲ bizarre behavior
   ▲ poor social functioning
   ▲ vague or unrealistic future plans
   ▲ depression
   ▲ phobias
   ▲ inability to cope with environment
   ▲ hopelessness
   ▲ growing inability to trust others
   ▲ increasing sense of isolation
   ▲ appearance of talking to himself or herself
   ▲ agitation
   ▲ looseness of association

Interventions

1. Complete primary and secondary survey with interventions, as indicated.
2. Assess for safety of patient, staff, and surrounding environment (e.g., waiting room).
3. Arrange for 1:1 observation if patient is a risk to him- or herself or others.
   ▲ Notify security per facility policy.
4. Use therapeutic communication at all times.
   ▲ Speak clearly, making one simple point at a time.
   ▲ Avoid threatening questions, including those that ask "why."
   ▲ Restate the person's statement to expand on his or her thought.
   ▲ Avoid making assumptions when reflecting back a patient's statement.
   ▲ Decrease the stimuli to the patient and promote a calm environment.
5. If patient is hearing voices, ask the patient what the voices are saying. Present the patient with reality by saying:
   ▲ "I can see you're really frightened, but I don't hear any voices."
   ▲ "Tell me, what do you hear them saying?"

Suicidal Behavior

▲ Suicide is the ninth leading cause of death in the United States.
  • It is the third leading cause of death among young people.
  • The highest rate of suicide occurs with those who are over the age of 65.
  • Every 16.8 minutes someone commits suicide.
▲ It is estimated that:
  • 775,000 Americans attempt suicide each year.
  • There is a 0.5% to 1% completion (death) rate among the nation's young.
  • There is a 25% completion rate among the nation's elderly.
  • There are 10 to 25 attempts for every (1) suicide completion.
  • Each suicide intimately affects at least six other people.
  • 57% of all suicide completions occur with a firearm.
▲ 75% of people who commit suicide send signals to those around them within 1 to 4 months before their death.
▲ Most people who attempt suicide are ambivalent about dying (NCIPC, 2002; Varcarolis, 1998).

 ALERT   Nurses **MUST** take every suicidal gesture seriously!

Assessment

A. Perform a general mental health assessment per protocol.
1. Associated information:
   - ▲ complete medical history and triage assessment
   - ▲ determine precipitating factors or events ("What makes today different?")
   - ▲ history of:
     - • substance abuse
     - • head trauma
     - • psychosis
     - • violent behavior
     - • schizophrenia
     - • aggression
     - • borderline personality
     - • organic diseases (e.g., temporal lobe epilepsy)
     - • depression
     - • abuse or assault
     - • suicidal ideation
     - • previous suicide attempts
     - • impulsivity
     - • family history of suicide
     - • chronic or disabling disease
2. Associated signs, symptoms, signals surrounding suicidal behavior:
   - ▲ giving possessions away
   - ▲ unusual peace or serenity
   - ▲ ambivalence
   - ▲ unnecessary risk taking
   - ▲ trouble sleeping
   - ▲ talk about death
   - ▲ refusal of basic essentials (food, meds, etc.)
   - ▲ lack of interest in personal hygiene
   - ▲ behavioral changes
   - ▲ increased use of drugs or alcohol
3. Age-specific considerations:
   - ▲ pediatric patients:
     - • unusual changes in behavior
       - − shy child becomes a thrill seeker
       - − outgoing child becomes withdrawn and disinterested
     - • giving possessions away
     - • sadness, despair, depression
     - • irritable or depressed moods
     - • victim of sexual, physical, or emotional abuse
     - • writes or draws pictures about death
   - ▲ adolescents:
     - • depression
     - • impulsive behavior
     - • trouble sleeping
     - • hopelessness
     - • rebellious behavior
     - • preoccupation with death
     - • suddenly seems happy after being sad for a long time
     - • conduct disorders
     - • social withdrawal from friends
     - • appetite disturbances
     - • helplessness
     - • chemical dependency
   - ▲ elderly patients:
     - • affective disorders
     - • decreased interest in food
     - • unusual safety risks
     - • early stages of dementia
       - − very high risk because they are aware of their growing deficits
     - • substance abuse
     - • misuse of prescribed medications
     - • refusal of medical interventions
4. High-risk factors for suicidal behavior:
   - ▲ adolescent
   - ▲ male
   - ▲ Caucasian
   - ▲ socially isolated
   - ▲ depression
   - ▲ hallucinations or delusions
   - ▲ intoxication
   - ▲ inadequate support system

▲ chronically or terminally ill
▲ has an established suicide plan
▲ prior suicide attempt
▲ high-risk professions:
  • physicians
  • police officers
  • attorneys
  • dentists
  • air-traffic controllers
  • military personnel
▲ older than 45 years

▲ separated, divorced, or widowed
▲ chemically dependent
▲ student
▲ coming out of a depressive state
▲ unemployed
▲ schizophrenic
▲ major life changes (job, family, etc.)
▲ major loss (health, spouse, etc.)
▲ intends shooting, hanging, jumping
▲ family history of suicide attempt

Interventions

1. Complete primary and secondary survey with interventions, as indicated.
2. Assess for patient safety and assign patient to treatment area as necessary.
3. Perform specific interventions based on injury inflicted (gunshot wound, ingestion, etc.).
4. Arrange for 1:1 observation.
5. Initiate crisis intervention.
6. Obtain lab work as ordered, including appropriate toxicology screens.
7. Treat the patient with sensitivity and respect (Box 2–7).
8. If you suspect that a depressed patient may be suicidal, ask:
   ▲ "Sometimes when people feel this depressed, hopeless, and/or sad, they have thoughts of hurting or killing themselves. Have you ever had thoughts like this?"
   ▲ If the patients answers "yes," then assess the following:
     • Does the person have a plan?
     • Assess lethality of plan (handful of aspirin versus a gun).
     • Does person have the means to carry out the plan?
     • Does the person have access to a gun, poison, car, etc.?
     • Has person ever attempted suicide before?
9. Conduct an environmental survey of the ED room in which the patient is being placed, and remove all unnecessary items from the room that may pose a risk to the patient's well-being including (but not limited to) gloves, extra linen, scalpels, gauze, and patient's clothing and belongings (patient should be in an exam gown).

> **! ALERT** Remember: You **MUST** take every suicidal gesture seriously!

■ Box 2–7: **DON'T LET THIS BE YOU**

She put on her new blue nightgown and combed her
  hair.
Painted her eyes and her mouth.
Used some Christmas cologne and then she
  swallowed the pills.

When they brought her to us,
Her gown was soiled and twisted around her body.
Her hair was damp and knotted.
The cosmetics grotesquely smeared on her tear-wet
  face.
She could still talk.
She took few enough pills for that:
"Let me alone, let me sleep."

We didn't have time to sympathize.
There was a man on the pacemaker in the next
  room.
A child had died an hour ago.
It was Sunday, too, and naturally we were short of
  help.
She was, frankly, a nuisance.

The resident passed the slender plastic tube
While she wept and fought, and we held her down.
The new nurse said, "Poor thing . . ."

I said, "Poor thing, nothing. If they're going to do it,
I wish they'd do it right and save us all this bother."
I didn't know she heard me. Maybe I didn't care.

That must have been a month ago.
Tonight she came in again,
D.O.A.
This time she'd hanged herself.
The way I knew her was the same blue nightgown—
  her face had changed.
The police found a note.
All it said was, "This time I'll do it right."

Only a couple of hours till midnight.
I'll be glad to finish up and go home.
I'm tired as usual and though it's warm in here,
I'm cold and not as unshaken as they think.
I know why I'm cold.
Death touched me again tonight.

Don't worry, I'm not going to brood about it.
It couldn't help her and I know it wouldn't me.
You can't go back.
You can't take back the words,
But I would if I could,
If only I could . . .
This once.

_____

(Author unknown)

OBSTETRIC ISSUES

General Issues

Common terms:
- ▲ Gravidity: Number of times a woman has been pregnant
- ▲ Parity: Number of pregnancies resulting in the birth of a viable fetus
- ▲ First trimester: First 12 weeks of pregnancy
- ▲ Second trimester: 13 to 26 weeks of pregnancy
- ▲ Third trimester: 12 weeks until delivery
- ▲ Precipitous birth: An imminent emergent delivery, occurs more often in multiparas
- ▲ Nuchal cord: The umbilical cord is wrapped around the infant's neck.

 Assessment

A. Obtain basic triage assessment per protocol.
B. Perform nursing assessment of the pregnant patient.
  1. Triage questions to ask:
- ▲ Do you feel the urge to push?
- ▲ How many babies have you had?
- ▲ Have the membranes ruptured?
  - • what color (green, clear)?
  - • gush of fluid?
  - • what time did it happen?
- ▲ Have you had any bright red discharge?
- ▲ How far apart are your contractions?
  - • how long does each one last?
- ▲ Is the baby crowning?
- ▲ Any heavy bleeding?
- ▲ Have you had any complications with your pregnancy?

  2. Signs and symptoms to assess for:
- ▲ nausea
- ▲ vomiting
- ▲ edema
- ▲ rectal pain
- ▲ fatigue
- ▲ fever
- ▲ syncope
- ▲ headache
- ▲ blurred vision
- ▲ sudden weight gain
- ▲ abdominal cramping
- ▲ hypertension

3. Past medical history:
   - ▲ cardiac disease
   - ▲ pulmonary disease
   - ▲ renal disease
   - ▲ hypertension
   - ▲ diabetes
   - ▲ thyroid disorders
   - ▲ seizure disorder
   - ▲ previous obstetric history
   - ▲ date of last normal menstrual cycle
   - ▲ estimated date of confinement
   - ▲ vaginal bleeding (color, amount, tissue)
   - ▲ chemical dependency
   - ▲ prenatal care

C. Auscultate for fetal heart tones (FHT):
   Using a fetal doppler, fetal heart rate can be assessed as early as 9 to 12 weeks' gestation. FHT can be detected by ultrasound at 6 to 8 weeks' gestation.
   1. Technique:
      - ▲ Using the doppler, locate and count the fetal heart rate.
      - ▲ Verify what the mother's heart rate is at that same time.
      - ▲ If the mother is having contractions:
        - • listen before the contraction to obtain a baseline FHT
        - • listen during the contraction
        - • listen 1 minute after the contraction finishes
   2. Interpretations of FHT:
      - ▲ Baseline rate is the average occurring between contractions.
        - • Normal is 120 to 160 beats per minute (bpm).
        - • Mild bradycardia is when the baseline rate is 100 to 119 bpm.
        - • Marked bradycardia is a baseline rate <99 bpm.
        - • Tachycardia is a persistent baseline rate >180 bpm.
          - – may occur with maternal fever, drug ingestion, thyrotoxicosis
          - – may occur with fetal infection or anemia

! ALERT   Marked bradycardia (fetal heart rate below 99 bpm) is cause for serious concern and immediate attention.

D. Time uterine contractions:
   1. Count from the beginning of one contraction to the beginning of the next contraction (as perceived by the mother or palpated by the nurse).
   2. Note how long each contraction lasts and the interval of the contractions.
   3. Count a series of contractions, since they may be irregularly spaced.

Spontaneous Abortion

▲ The termination of pregnancy before fetal viability
▲ Delivery of the fetus before 20 weeks' gestation
▲ General population freely uses the term *abortion* to indicate one that is an induced abortion.
▲ *Miscarriage* is the term used by the general population to indicate a spontaneous abortion.
  • Health care personnel should be sensitive to the layperson's use of terms. Refrain from telling a grieving mother that she just had a "spontaneous abortion"—instead, use the term "miscarriage."
▲ Parents should be counseled regarding their loss and the grieving that will take place.
▲ Six classifications are listed in Table 2–19.

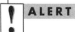

Interventions

1. Dependent on type of loss
2. May need IV access for administration of fluids and/or medications
3. Rh coagulation profile (administration of RhoGAM if woman is Rh negative)
4. Provide emotional care for grieving woman and family.

Ectopic Pregnancy

▲ The implantation of the fertilized ovum outside the uterine cavity
  • 96% of ectopic implantations occur in the fallopian tubes

> **! ALERT**   Vaginal bleeding and abdominal pain in a reproductive-age female signify an ectopic pregnancy **until proven otherwise.**

Assessment

1. History:
   ▲ pelvic inflammatory disease (PID)
   ▲ congenital or developmental anomalies of the fallopian tube(s)
   ▲ previous ectopic pregnancy
   ▲ tubal ligation
   ▲ use of an intrauterine device
   ▲ infertility
   ▲ multiple induced abortions
   ▲ endometriosis

TABLE 2–19 • Spontaneous Abortions

Type	Sign and Symptoms	Uterine Cramping	Bleeding	Passage of Tissue	Internal Cervical Os	Possible Management
Threatened	Low back pain Uterine tenderness	Menstrual-like cramps	Slight	No	Closed	Bed rest
Inevitable	Uterus enlarged and boggy	Moderate	Moderate	No	Open	D & C
Incomplete	Possible hypovolemic shock Uterus enlarged and boggy Uterus smaller than expected for dates	Severe	Heavy	Yes	Open, with tissue in the os	D & C
Complete	Uterus small and non-tender	Mild	Scant	Yes	Closed	Variable
Septic	Fever Malodorous vaginal bleeding Uterus extremely tender upon palpation	Variable	Variable	Variable	Open	D & C Antibiotics Maintain ABCs
Missed	History of missed menses Uterus smaller than expected for dates Ultrasound shows intrauterine products of conception without heartbeat	No	Slight	No	Closed	Fetal delivery

2. Common signs and symptoms:
   - ▲ sudden, unilateral, severe pelvic pain
   - ▲ nausea and vomiting
   - ▲ syncope
   - ▲ cervical motion tenderness
   - ▲ enlarged uterus
   - ▲ amenorrhea (average, 5.5 weeks)
   - ▲ 1 to 2 days of abnormal vaginal spotting
   - ▲ positive orthostatic vital signs
   - ▲ abdominal pain on palpation
   - ▲ tachycardia and hypotension
3. Abnormal lab values:
   - ▲ WBC elevated
   - ▲ serum quantitative B-hCG
   - ▲ decreased hemoglobin and hematocrit

Interventions

1. Maintain ABCs.
2. Monitor vital signs closely.
3. Place one or two large-bore IV lines; rate depends on hemodynamic status.
4. Type and cross as indicated for transfusion.
5. Provide patient support and education for loss of pregnancy and preoperative preparation.
6. Administer Rh immunoglobulin to all Rh-negative patients.

▶ *Placenta Previa*

Placenta is abnormally implanted in the lower uterine segment, to some degree occluding the cervical os.

 Assessment

1. Common signs and symptoms:
   - ▲ PAINLESS vaginal bleeding occurring at 28 to 32 weeks' gestation
   - ▲ bright red vaginal bleeding
   - ▲ FHTs may show ominous patterns
   - ▲ ultrasound shows placenta over cervical os

 Interventions

1. *Do not perform a vaginal examination;* it can cause fatal hemorrhage.
2. Maintain ABCs.
3. Position mother on her left side (displaces the uterus off the inferior vena cava).
4. Type and cross as indicated for transfusion.
5. Establish and maintain large-bore IV line(s).
6. Monitor vital signs of mother and fetal heart tones closely.
7. Assess CBC, coagulation studies, and Rh antibody status.

 ALERT — Painless vaginal bleeding in a pregnant woman is significant for the risk of placenta previa—do NOT perform a vaginal examination since it may cause fetal hemorrhage!

▶ *Abruptio Placentae*

Accidental hemorrhage caused by the separation of the normally located placenta before delivery of the fetus.

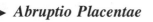

Assessment

1. History:
   - ▲ essential hypertension
   - ▲ multiple gestation
   - ▲ external trauma
   - ▲ smoking
   - ▲ uterine fibroids
   - ▲ pregnancy-induced hypertension
   - ▲ previous abruptio placentae or placenta previa
   - ▲ substance abuse (especially cocaine)
   - ▲ preterm premature rupture of membranes
   - ▲ advanced maternal age
2. Common signs and symptoms:
   - ▲ tender, rigid uterus
   - ▲ fetal distress
   - ▲ **PAINFUL** vaginal bleeding
   - ▲ vaginal bleeding may be absent
     - • if encapsulated by placenta or membranes
3. Complications:
   - ▲ fetal death
   - ▲ renal failure
   - ▲ hypovolemic shock
   - ▲ disseminated intravascular coagulation (DIC)

Interventions

1. Maintain ABCs.
2. Do not perform a vaginal examination until placenta previa is ruled out.
3. Monitor maternal vital signs and fetal heart rate closely.
4. Place large-bore IV line(s).
5. Position mother on her left side (displaces uterus off the inferior vena cava).
6. Type and cross as indicated for transfusion.
7. Assess CBC, Rh status, coagulation studies, toxicology screen.
8. Prepare for possibility of emergency delivery.

 ALERT Painful vaginal bleeding in a pregnant woman is significant for the risk of abruptio placentae.

Pre-eclampsia and Eclampsia

These complications of pregnancy-induced hypertension are the leading cause of maternal death in the United States.

 Assessment

1. Characteristic symptoms:
   - ▲ onset of symptoms from the 20th week of gestation to 1 to 10 days' postpartum
   - ▲ hypertension
     - if positive pregestational history of hypertension, compare current BP with patient's normal BP
     - if negative history of pregestional hypertension, then hypertension is considered anything above a systolic BP >120 or diastolic BP >80 to 90 mmHg
   - ▲ proteinuria (300 mg or more of protein excreted in a 24-hour period)
   - ▲ nondependent edema, present after 8 to 12 hours of bed rest (face, fingers, body)
   - ▲ weight gain >2 lb in 1 week, or 6 lb in 1 month
2. *Severe* pre-eclampsia will have additional symptoms:
   - ▲ systolic BP >160 mmHg
   - ▲ oliguria
   - ▲ severe headache
   - ▲ pulmonary edema
   - ▲ hyperreflexia
   - ▲ serum creatinine >1.2 mg/dl
   - ▲ retinal hemorrhages
   - ▲ decreased fibrinogen level
   - ▲ diastolic BP >110 mmHg
   - ▲ proteinuria (>5 g/24-hr sample)
   - ▲ visual changes (blurring, double vision)
   - ▲ thrombocytopenia (platelet count <100,000)
   - ▲ intrauterine growth retardation
   - ▲ increased liver enzymes
   - ▲ papilledema
   - ▲ epigastric pain (indicative of hepatic hemorrhage)
3. Eclampsia occurs when the central nervous system is so influenced by vasospasm that seizures develop.

Interventions (depend on the severity of the disease and symptoms)

1. Maintain ABCs.
2. Monitor maternal vital signs and FHT closely.
3. Establish IV access site(s) for medication administration.
4. Initiate a conservative rate with crystalloid fluid rate *no greater than* 100 mL/hr.

5. Strictly record intake and output.
6. Place Foley catheter.
7. Administer magnesium sulfate (MgSO$_4$) to prevent and treat convulsions.
   - ▲ Loading dose of 3 to 4 g
   - ▲ Continual MgSO$_4$ IV drip dose of 1 to 4 g/hr
   - ▲ May be given IM if IV access not immediately available.
8. Prepare for immediate delivery if patient's condition worsens.

Gestational Diabetes Mellitus

May occur in previously nondiabetic women as a result of metabolic changes.

 Assessment

1. History:
   - ▲ stillbirth
   - ▲ hydramnios
   - ▲ maternal obesity
   - ▲ hypertension
   - ▲ infant with congenital anomalies
   - ▲ infant weight >9 lbs
   - ▲ family history of diabetes
   - ▲ maternal age >35
2. Effects of diabetes on:
   - ▲ mother
     - increased risk of pregnancy-induced hypertension
     - infections that may be more severe
     - birth trauma owing to increased fetal size
     - postpartum hemorrhage
   - ▲ fetus
     - faulty DNA and RNA synthesis, resulting in congenital anomalies
     - delayed lung maturity
     - increased fetal growth rate
     - after birth, neonatal hypoglycemia
3. Common symptoms:
   - ▲ polyuria
   - ▲ polydipsia
   - ▲ glucosuria
   - ▲ chronic monilial infection
   - ▲ polyphagia
   - ▲ weight loss
   - ▲ urine positive for ketones

4. Laboratory values:
   ▲ elevated serum glucose levels at 24 to 28 weeks (>125 mg/dl)
   ▲ elevated serum glucose challenge test

 Interventions

1. Stabilize serum glucose level.
2. Provide patient education, including:
   ▲ facts about gestational diabetes
   ▲ nutritional counseling
   ▲ exercise
3. Close follow-up with primary care provider if patient is discharged.

Premature Rupture of Membranes

The spontaneous rupture of amniotic membranes before the onset of labor regardless of gestational age

 Assessment

1. History:
   ▲ multiple gestations
   ▲ breech presentations
   ▲ chorioamnionitis
   ▲ fetal distress
2. Common signs and symptoms:
   ▲ fluid from vagina, in varying amounts
3. Complications:
   ▲ amnionitis
   ▲ endometritis
   ▲ asphyxia
   ▲ prematurity
   ▲ cord prolapse
   ▲ fetal injuries secondary to low amniotic fluid volume
   ▲ malpresentation
   ▲ respiratory distress
   ▲ cord compression

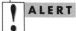 **ALERT**   Treatment of premature rupture of the membranes depends on the gestational age of the fetus and if the woman's labor has begun.

Interventions

1. Monitor vitals signs and FHR.
2. Perform sterile speculum exam.
   ▲ Assess for cervical effacement and dilation.
   ▲ Evaluate fluid from the posterior vaginal vault using litmus or nitrazine paper.
     • amniotic fluid is alkaline and will turn litmus or nitrazine paper blue
     • blood can give a false-positive nitrazine test
     • microscopic evaluation of dried fluid for a ferning pattern
     • blood or other secretions can produce a false-negative ferning test
   ▲ If fluid leakage is intermittent, nitrazine, litmus, and ferning exams may be inconclusive for intact membranes.
   ▲ Evaluate for a prolapsed umbilical cord.
3. Defer bimanual examination until labor is active.
4. Establish and maintain large-bore IV line(s).

▶ *Preterm Labor*

Occurs at 20 to 37 weeks' gestation and produces cervical changes

Assessment

1. History
   ▲ infection
   ▲ fetal abnormalities
   ▲ multiple gestation
   ▲ cerclage
   ▲ cocaine use
   ▲ abortion
   ▲ trauma
   ▲ poor nutritional status
   ▲ emotional stress
   ▲ maternal fever or sepsis
   ▲ maternal diabetes
   ▲ diethylstilbestrol (DES) exposure in utero
     • DES causes cervical anomalies and incompetence
   ▲ uterine anomalies
   ▲ previous cervical conization
   ▲ previous preterm birth
   ▲ abdominal surgery during this pregnancy
   ▲ maternal age <18 years or >35 years
   ▲ absent or inadequate prenatal care

- ▲ more than 10 cigarettes smoked in a day
- ▲ second- or third-trimester bleeding
2. Common signs and symptoms:
   - ▲ menstrual cramps
   - ▲ back discomfort
   - ▲ vaginal pain
   - ▲ abdominal pain or discomfort
   - ▲ change in vaginal discharge
   - ▲ pelvic, rectal, or bladder pressure

 Interventions

1. Monitor maternal vital signs and FHR.
2. Time several contractions, when possible.
3. Perform sterile speculum exam, as stated for PROM.
4. Perform gentle bimanual exam if membranes *are not* ruptured.
5. Establish large-bore IV line(s).
6. Arrange for transfer to labor and delivery unit and for fetal monitoring.

Trauma in Pregnancy

- ▲ Fetal survival depends on the integrity of the woman's condition and stability.
- ▲ Initially, all efforts should be centered on stabilization and treatment of the woman, with subsequent evaluation and treatment of the unborn child.

Assessment

1. History:
   - ▲ fall
   - ▲ physical assault
   - ▲ motor vehicle crash
2. Primary and secondary assessments as indicated for *all* trauma victims.
3. Uterine activity, including:
   - ▲ tenderness or contractions
   - ▲ cervical dilation
   - ▲ vaginal bleeding
   - ▲ umbilical cord prolapse
   - ▲ ruptured membranes
4. Fetal distress:
   - ▲ fetal heart tones
   - ▲ fetal movement
   - ▲ fetal monitoring

Interventions

1. Maintain ABCs.
2. Immobilize the c-spine.
3. Refer to Multiple Trauma Guideline.
4. If no c-spine injury, place woman on her left side to prevent inferior vena cava compression and hypotension.
   - ▲ If woman has a spinal injury, log-roll patient on the spinal board and support board with rolled towels under it, to maintain patient on her left side.
5. Anticipate hypovolemia and treat blood loss aggressively.
6. CT scans are often suggested, since plain films of the abdomen may be distorted.
7. A pediatrician and an obstetrician should be mobilized to the ED for evaluation and preparation for possible emergency delivery.
8. Administer tetanus prophylaxis per protocol.
9. Transfer to obstetric unit on stabilization.

► *Precipitous or Emergency Delivery*

- ▲ Optimally, childbirth should occur in the labor and delivery department of a hospital. On rare occasions, however, a woman will deliver before arriving in the obstetric department.
- ▲ The ED staff must be prepared to care for the mother and baby in this situation.

Assessment

1. Signs of imminent delivery:
   - ▲ increased bloody show
   - ▲ contractions every 2 to 3 minutes
   - ▲ involuntary pushing
   - ▲ perineal and rectal flattening
   - ▲ crowning of the fetal scalp at the introitus
   - ▲ rectal pressure or passage of feces
   - ▲ mother states "the baby is coming"
   - ▲ spontaneous rupture of membranes
   - ▲ bulging of the perineum

 ALERT If delivery is imminent, do *NOT* attempt to transport the patient. Prepare for a controlled delivery in the ED.

Interventions

1. Obtain necessary equipment:
   - ▲ **emergent birth kit** that includes:
     - small sterile drape
     - 2 sterile Kelly clamps
     - 2 umbilical cord clamps
     - infant blanket
     - bulb syringe
     - sterile scissors
     - sterile gloves
   - ▲ protective gloves, masks, gowns
   - ▲ neonatal resuscitative equipment
   - ▲ ample linen
   - ▲ wall or portable suction
2. Obtain isolette or warmed blankets for newborn.
3. Continually care for the mother until delivery of the placenta; observe for hemorrhage.
4. Assess Apgar score for infant at 1 and 5 minutes (Table 2–20).
5. Document important information:
   - ▲ time of membrane rupture
   - ▲ time of birth
   - ▲ type of presentation
   - ▲ cord around neck?
   - ▲ time of placenta delivery
   - ▲ Apgar scores at 1 and 5 minutes

TABLE 2–20 • Apgar Scoring Chart

	Sign	0	1	2	1-minute Score	5-minute Score
A	**Appearance** (color)	Blue or pale	Pink body with blue extremities	Completely pink		
P	**Pulse** (heart rate)	Absent	Slow (<100)	Greater than 100		
G	**Grimace** (reflexes)	No response	Facial grimace	Cough, sneeze, crying		
A	**Activity** (muscle tone)	Limp	Some flexion	Active motion		
R	**Respirations**	Absent	Slow, irregular (weak cry)	Good (vigorous crying)		

ORTHOPEDIC INJURIES

General Issues

Assessment

A. Obtain and record triage assessment:
  - ▲ mechanism of injury
  - ▲ time of injury
  - ▲ immediate care of injured extremity
    - • splinted
    - • ice applied
    - • elevated
    - • walked on it
  - ▲ possibility of other injuries
B. Assess injured area for:
  - ▲ obvious deformity
    - • angulation
    - • rotation
    - • shortening
  - ▲ swelling
  - ▲ pain
    - • at rest
    - • with movement
    - • on palpation
    - • point tenderness
  - ▲ decreased sensation
  - ▲ partial or complete loss of motor function
  - ▲ change in skin temperature
  - ▲ blanching of the area
  - ▲ quality of pulses distal to the injury
C. Complete remainder of basic triage assessment and **document** accurately.

Immediate Care If

- ▲ Open fracture:
  - • Notify ED physician immediately.
  - • Aseptically control bleeding.
  - • Assess for signs of infection.
  - • Cover open wound with sterile gauze.
  - • Arrange for stabilization of the injury.

▲ Closed fracture that:
  • is unstable
  • creates alteration in circulation distal to injury
▲ Advise ED physician of patient status.

 Interventions

1. Remove *all* rings from *all* fingers with hand, wrist, or forearm injuries.
2. If closed injury with possibility of a fracture:
   ▲ reassure patient
   ▲ apply splint to increase patient comfort and decrease risk of further injury
   ▲ apply ice and elevate extremity

3. If triage nurse anticipates the need for an x-ray:
   ▲ follow departmental policy with regard to ordering x-ray study from triage

▶ *Other Presentations*

See Figure 2–3.

▲ Common pediatric fractures (Salter-Harris Fractures; Table 2–21)
  • The growth plates in the bones of children are weaker than nearby ligaments.
  • When an injury occurs, the ligaments hold tight, and a fracture of the growth plate results.
  • These fractures are easily missed on x–ray and should be treated based on history and clinical presentation (Molczan, 2001).
▲ Reflex sympathetic dystrophy
  • A syndrome that is characterized by extreme pain, loss of function, and evidence of sympathetic imbalance
  • This syndrome is also known as causalgia and complex regional pain syndrome.
  • Irritation of the sympathetic peripheral nerves causes abnormal sympathetic function, resulting in circulatory changes, swelling, and burning pain (Mutch, 2001).
▲ Nursemaid's elbow in children
  • Results from a "pull" injury to the annular ligament that surrounds the radial head at the elbow
  • Very common in children ages 1 to 5 years
  • There is minimal pain on palpation and little swelling; however, the child refuses to use the arm.
    – parents often present with their child, believing there is a wrist injury
    – child won't move the arm or the hand, holding the elbow motionless at the side or waist

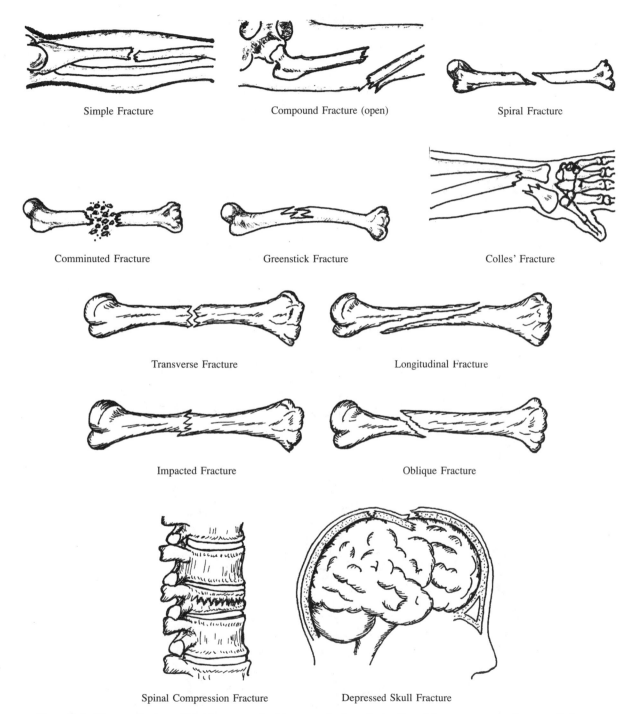

Simple Fracture

Compound Fracture (open)

Spiral Fracture

Comminuted Fracture

Greenstick Fracture

Colles' Fracture

Transverse Fracture

Longitudinal Fracture

Impacted Fracture

Oblique Fracture

Spinal Compression Fracture

Depressed Skull Fracture

Figure 2–3. Common fractures, The triage nurse should posses a basic understanding of the most common fractures. Doing so enhances the nurse's ability to prioritize the patient's acuity and provide initial nursing care of the patient.

TABLE 2-21 • Salter-Harris Fractures

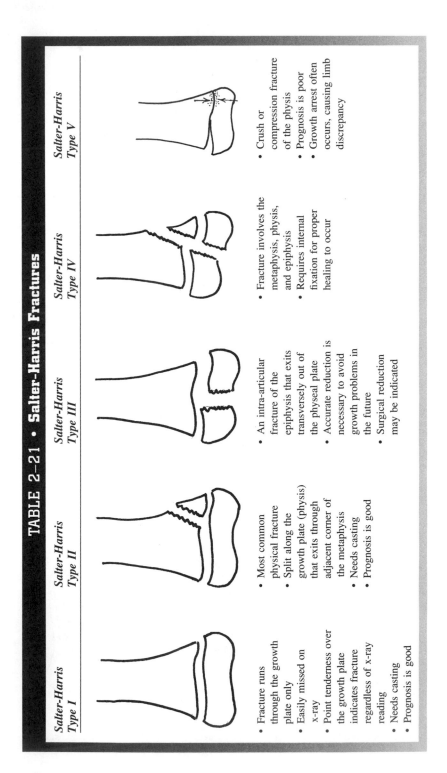

Salter-Harris Type I	Salter-Harris Type II	Salter-Harris Type III	Salter-Harris Type IV	Salter-Harris Type V
• Fracture runs through the growth plate only • Easily missed on x-ray • Point tenderness over the growth plate indicates fracture regardless of x-ray reading • Needs casting • Prognosis is good	• Most common physical fracture • Split along the growth plate (physis) that exits through adjacent corner of the metaphysis • Needs casting • Prognosis is good	• An intra-articular fracture of the epiphysis that exits transversely out of the physeal plate • Accurate reduction is necessary to avoid growth problems in the future • Surgical reduction may be indicated	• Fracture involves the metaphysis, physis, and epiphysis • Requires internal fixation for proper healing to occur	• Crush or compression fracture of the physis • Prognosis is poor • Growth arrest often occurs, causing limb discrepancy

POISONINGS

▲ May occur intentionally or accidentally
▲ Patients may present stating what the substance was, or may have no idea what it was that has made them so ill (Table 2–22).

Assessment

A. Complete a basic triage assessment.
B. Perform a subjective and objective assessment for risk of poisoning.
   1. Neurologic
      ▲ lethargy
      ▲ agitation
      ▲ coma
      ▲ hallucinations
      ▲ seizures
   2. Respiratory
      ▲ respiratory depression
      ▲ poor airway control
   3. Cardiovascular
      ▲ tachycardia
      ▲ arrhythmias
      ▲ torsades de pointes
      ▲ hypotension
      ▲ hypertension
   4. Vital signs
      ▲ hyperthermia
      ▲ hypothermia
      ▲ tachycardia
      ▲ bradycardia
      ▲ hypertension
      ▲ hypotension

Interventions

1. Maintain ABCs.
2. Nursing care will vary depending on the poisoning substance.

TABLE 2-22 • Poisonings

Substance and Common/Street Name	Clinical Signs and Symptoms
ACETAMINOPHEN Tylenol	Nausea, vomiting, anorexia, malaise, oliguria, increased liver enzymes Diffuse abdominal pain which becomes right upper-quadrant abdominal pain
ALCOHOL	Sedation, relaxation, euphoria, memory loss, poor judgment, ataxia, slurred speech, nausea, vomiting, obtundation, coma In children, hypoglycemia occurs
AMPHETAMINE Prescription: Ritalin, Tenuate, Preludin, Dexedrine Street: ice, crank, cat, jeff, ecstasy, mulka, crystal, speed	CNS: agitation, delirium, hyperactivity, tremors, dizziness, mydriasis, CVA, headache, hyperreflexia, seizures, coma Psychiatric: euphoria, aggressive behavior, anxiety, hallucinations, compulsive repetitious actions Cardiopulmonary: palpitations, hypertensive crisis, tachycardia, reflex bradycardia, dysrhythmias, myocardial infarction, aortic dissection, pulmonary edema, respiratory distress
ANTICHOLINERGIC antihistamines, antiparkinsonian, cyclic antidepressants, antipsychotics, antispasmodics, mushrooms, jimsonweed	**Classic toxidrome:** "Mad as a hatter"—altered mental status "Hot as a hare"—hyperthermia "Red as a beet"—flushed skin "Dry as a bone"—dry skin and mucous membranes "Blind as a bat"—blurred vision secondary to mydriasis (Rosen, 1999)
ARSENIC	Acute ingestion: severe hemorrhagic gastroenteritis develops within hours, bone marrow depression, encephalopathy, cardiomyopathy, pulmonary edema, cardiac dysrhythmia, peripheral neuropathy Chronic ingestion: weakness, anorexia, hyperkeratosis, hyperpigmentation, hepatic injury, respiratory irritation, perforated nasal septum, tremor, peripheral neuropathy
BARBITURATE Pentothal, Nembutal, Seconal, Mysoline, Phenobarbital	CNS: lethargy, slurred speech, incoordination, ataxia, coma, hyporeflexia, nystagmus, stupor Cardiopulmonary: hypotension, bradycardia, respiratory depression, apnea Other: rhabdomyolysis, compartment syndrome, hypoglycemia
BENZODIAZEPINE Xanax, Librium, Clonopin, Valium, Dalmane, Ativan, Versed, Serax, Restoril, Halcion	CNS: nystagmus, miosis, diplopia, impaired speech and coordination, amnesia, ataxia, confusion, somnolence, depressed deep-endon reflexes, dyskinesia Cardiopulmonary. hypotension, bradycardia, tachycardia (in response to the hypotension), respiratory depression, aspiration Other: hypothermia, rhabdomyolysis, skin necrosis
BETA BLOCKER atenolol, Brevibloc, Inderal, Lopressor, Tenormin, Timoptic	CNS: seizures, coma, CNS depression Cardiopulmonary: hypotension, bradycardia, cardiac conduction delays, heart block, heart failure, bronchospasm, pulmonary edema, respiratory depression

TABLE 2–22 • Poisonings (Continued)

Substance and Common/Street Name	Clinical Signs and Symptoms
CALCIUM CHANNEL BLOCKER Cardizem, Procardia, Calan SR	CNS: syncope, CNS depression, rare seizure, coma Cardiopulmonary: severe bradycardia, atrioventricular block, intraventricular conduction delays, ventricular dysrhythmias, congestive heart failure, respiratory depression, pulmonary edema Other: hyperglycemia, nausea, vomiting, ileus, hypotension, metabolic acidosis
CARBAMAZEPINE Oral antiseizure medication with a structure similar to tricyclic antidepressants	CNS: ataxia, dizziness, drowsiness, nystagmus, hallucinations, combativeness, coma, seizures Cardiopulmonary: respiratory depression, aspiration pneumonia, hypotension, conduction, disturbances, supraventricular tachycardia, bradycardia, ECG changes Other: urinary retention, hyponatremia, myoclonus
CARBON MONOXIDE	CNS: headache, dizziness, ataxia, confusion, acute encephalopathy, syncope, seizures, coma Cardiopulmonary: chest pain, palpitations, dyspnea, myocardial infarction, tachycardia, hypotension Other: nausea, vomiting, decreased vision, retinal hemorrhage, lactic acidosis, rhabdomyolysis
CHLORAL HYDRATE	CNS: headache, lightheadedness, ataxia, hyporeflexia, altered mental status Cardiopulmonary: hypotension, ventricular and supraventricular dysrhythmias, bradypnea Other: nausea, vomiting, abdominal pain, rash, pearlike breath odor
CYANIDE	CNS: headache, confusion, syncope, seizures, coma, agitation, CNS stimulation Cardiopulmonary: tachycardia and hypertension progress into bradycardia and hypotension
DIGOXIN	CNS: colored visual halos, blurred vision, agitation, lethargy, seizures, psychosis, hallucinations Cardiopulmonary: hypotension, cardiovascular collapse, bradycardia, AV block, PAT, CHF Other: nausea, vomiting, diarrhea, abdominal pain
ETHYLENE GLYCOL	CNS: ataxia, slurred speech, irritability, cerebral edema, convulsions, coma Cardiopulmonary: tachycardia, bradycardia, hypotension, hypertension, pulmonary edema Other: nausea, vomiting, abdominal pain, hematemesis, acute renal failure, myalgia, hypocalcemia
HALLUCINOGEN	CNS: restlessness, anxiety, incipient dread, distortions of reality, helplessness, coma, hyperreflexia Cardiopulmonary: tachycardia, hypertension, dysrhythmias, tachypnea, respiratory arrest Other: nausea, vomiting, hyperpyrexia, coagulopathies

TABLE 2-22 • Poisonings (Continued)

Substance and Common/Street Name	Clinical Signs and Symptoms
HYDROCARBON	CNS: intoxication, headache, euphoria, slurred speech, lethargy, coma Cardiopulmonary: respiratory distress, cyanosis, aspiration, tachycardia, dysrhythmia Other: mucosal irritation, gastritis, diarrhea, acute renal failure
HYPOGLYCEMIC AGENT	CNS: headache, blurred vision, anxiety, irritability, confusion, stupor, coma, seizures Cardiopulmonary: respiratory distress, apnea, palpitations, tachycardia, hypertension, PVCs Other: nausea, facial flushing, hypoglycemia, pallor
IRON	CNS: lethargy, seizures, coma Cardiopulmonary: tachycardia, tachypnea, hypotension, Other: vomiting, abdominal pain, GI bleeding, diarrhea, renal failure, hepatic necrosis
ISONIAZID	CNS: ataxia, hyperreflexia, agitation, hallucinations, psychosis, coma, seizures Cardiopulmonary: hypotension, tachycardia, shock, respiratory depression, Kussmaul respirations Other: hyperthermia, nausea, vomiting, severe anion gap, phabdomyolysis
LEAD (ADULT)	CNS: headache, confusion, altered mental status, seizures, nerve entrapment, motor neuropathy Cardiopulmonary/reproductive: hypertension, alteration in sperm count and quality Other: anorexia, dyspepsia, constipation, renal failure
LEAD (PEDIATRIC)	CNS: cognitive dysfunction, decreased IQ, encephalopathy, irritability, headache, coma Hematologic: anemia, basophilic stippling Other: nausea, vomiting, abdominal pain, mild hearing loss
LITHIUM	CNS: lethargy, confusion, tremor, ataxia, slurred speech, hyperreflexia, clonus, dystonia Cardiopulmonary: ECG changes, respiratory failure Other: nausea, vomiting, diarrhea, diabetes insipidus, leukocytosis
METHANOL	CNS: inebriation, ataxia, seizures, coma, blurred vision, dilated pupils, headache, confusion Cardiopulmonary: hyperpnea, hypotension Other: metabolic acidosis, nausea, vomiting, abdominal pain

TABLE 2–22 • Poisonings (Continued)

Substance and Common/Street Name	Clinical Signs and Symptoms
NONSTEROIDAL ANTI-INFLAMMATORIES	CNS: drowsiness, dizziness, lethargy, seizures Cardiopulmonary: hypotension, tachycardia, hyperventilation, apnea Other: nausea, vomiting, abdominal pain, acute renal failure, metabolic acidosis
ORGANOPHOSPHATE	CNS: headache, dizziness, tremors, anxiety, weakness, incoordination, convulsions, coma Cardiopulmonary: hypotension, bradycardia, AV block, asystole, bronchospasm, pulmonary edema Other: miosis, anorexia, abdominal cramps, salivation, lacrimation
PHENCYCLIDINE	CNS: impaired judgment, agitation, violent behavior, psychosis, paranoia, coma, seizures, dyskinesia Cardiopulmonary: hypertension, tachycardia, apnea Other: hyperthermia, acute renal failure, hypoglycemia
PHENOTHIAZINE	CNS: agitation, seizures, coma, extrapyramidal signs, tardive dyskinesia Cardiopulmonary: respiratory depression, pulmonary edema, tachycardia, ECG changes, V tach Other: hyperthermia, priapism, acute renal failure, constipation, ileus, agranulocytosis, anemia
PHENYTOIN	CNS: ataxia, nystagmus, cortical depression, confusion, slurred speech, coma, seizures Cardiopulmonary: hypotension, bradycardia, myocardial depression with rapid IV infusion Other: nausea, vomiting
SALICYLATE	CNS: tinnitus, deafness, delirium, seizures, coma, agitation, lethargy, confusion, cerebral edema Cardiopulmonary: hypotension, shock, tachypnea, noncardiac pulmonary edema, hyperventilation Other: nausea, vomiting, hepatic injury, acute renal insufficiency, hematemesis
SYMPATHOMIMETIC	CNS: anxiety, headache, agitation, altered mentation, diaphoresis, stroke, seizures Cardiopulmonary: palpitations, chest pain, myocardial ischemia, tachydysrhythmias, hypertension Other: dilated pupils, dry mucous membranes, urinary retention, hyperthermia
THEOPHYLLINE	CNS: tremor, agitation, nervousness, seizures Cardiopulmonary: hypotension, tachycardia, tachypnea, hypertension, dysrhythmias Other: nausea, vomiting, abdominal pain, hypokalemia, hyperglycemia, leukocytosis

TABLE 2-22 • Poisonings (Continued)

Substance and Common/Street Name	Clinical Signs and Symptoms
TOLUENE	CNS: depression, euphoria, ataxia, seizures, insomnia, headache, coma Cardiopulmonary: sudden cardiac death, dilated cardiomyopathy, myocardial infarction Other: renal failure, rhabdomyolysis, hematemesis, abdominal pain
TRICYCLIC ANTIDEPRESSANT	CNS: agitation, tremors, seizures, drowsiness, lethargy, coma, ataxia, mania, dilated pupils Cardiopulmonary: hypotension, tachycardia, bradycardia, ECG changes, dysrhythmias Other: urinary retention, priapism, leukopenia, nausea, vomiting

(Rosen, 1999; Dart, 2000)

▶ RASH

- ▲ A broad term used to describe a dermatologic manifestation that may include:
  - hives
  - infections (fungal, viral, bacterial)
  - insect bites
  - contact dermatitis
  - folliculitis
- ▲ Rashes may be:
  - primary
  - secondary
  - vascular
  - contagious
- ▲ It is *vital* for the nurse to be able to properly document the lesions and to identify those that may be contagious.
- ▲ When inspecting the skin, be sure to have:
  - adequate lighting
  - tape measure to assist in assessing the size of the lesions.
- ▲ Patient privacy should be maintained during this evaluation.
- ▲ Always wear gloves when assessing a rash or skin lesion.

▶ *General Issues*

Assessment

A. Obtain and record triage assessment:
  1. History of allergies:
     - ▲ prior exposures, reactions, or anaphylaxis
     - ▲ new products or medications
  2. Characteristics of rash:
     - ▲ location
       - localized
       - widespread
       - area of the body
     - ▲ size
       - approximate size of lesions
     - ▲ shape
       - linear
       - circular
       - grouped
       - scattered

- generalized
- diffuse
▲ color
  - pink
  - red
  - purple
  - yellow
  - brown
  - green
▲ consistency
  - flat or smooth
  - raised or bumpy
  - hard or soft
  - firm
▲ temperature
  - cool
  - warm
  - hot to touch
▲ mobility
  - fixed
  - movable masses
  - fluid filled
  - open
  - draining
▲ signs of infection
  - redness
  - swelling
  - red streaks
  - warm to touch

3. Associated symptoms and behavior:
   ▲ fever
   ▲ headache
   ▲ drowsiness
   ▲ facial or eye swelling
   ▲ "cold" symptoms
   ▲ itching
   ▲ sore throat
   ▲ joint pain
   ▲ vision changes
   ▲ refusal or inability to swallow
   ▲ nausea, vomiting, or diarrhea
   ▲ swollen glands

B. Assess for risk factors that may increase the acuity of a rash:
   ▲ prior allergic reaction
   ▲ chronic illness

▲ immunosuppressed
  • congenital
  • acquired
  • chemically induced

 Immediate Care If

▲ Difficulty breathing, wheezing, and/or chest tightness
▲ Recent exposure to possible or known toxin with development of:
  • cough
  • slurred speech
  • hoarseness
  • swollen tongue
  • difficulty swallowing
▲ Wheezing after:
  • ingestion of medication
  • exposure to an allergic food
  • bee sting
▲ Purple or blood-colored spots with or without a fever
▲ Fever greater than 105°F
▲ Bright red skin that peels off in sheets
▲ Severe headache with a fever >100°F
▲ Hives began <2 hours ago and patient has had severe allergic reaction in the past

 ALERT   Use prescribed anaphylactic kit as directed for known allergies.

◤ *Primary Lesions*

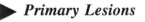 **Assessment**

▲ Primary lesions arise from previously normal skin (Figure 2–4):
  • macule = flat, nonpalpable, discolored, <1 cm
    – freckle
    – drug rash
    – measles
    – scarlet fever
  • papule = elevated, solid lesion <1 cm
    – wart
    – raised scaly area of psoriasis

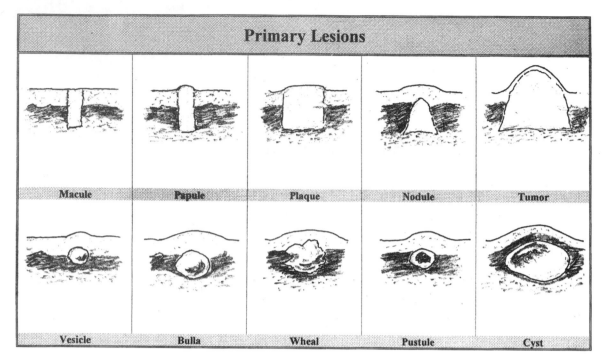

Figure 2–4. Primary lesions.

  - small bug bite
  - pityriasis rosea
- plaque = like a macule or papule, but >1 cm in diameter
  - birthmark
  - mongolian spot
  - plantar wart
  - psoriasis
  - pityriasis rosea
- nodule = elevated, solid lesion 1 to 2 cm in diameter, moves with skin when palpated
  - ganglion
  - area of poorly absorbed injection
- tumor = elevated, solid lesion >2 cm, may be soft or firm
  - tumor of any type
- vesicle = elevated lesion <1 cm filled with clear fluid
  - blister
  - chickenpox
  - poison ivy
  - herpes simplex
  - herpes zoster

- bulla = elevated lesion >1 cm, filled with clear fluid
  - bullous impetigo
  - syphilis
  - poison ivy
  - burns
- pustule = elevated, pus-filled lesion
  - acne
  - impetigo
  - boil
- wheal = elevated lesion, with circumscribed pink borders and light center
  - hives
  - urticaria
  - insect bite
  - poison sumac
  - poison ivy
- cyst = encapsulated, fluid-filled area in the dermis or subcutaneous tissue
  - sebaceous cyst
  - epidermoid cyst

▶ *Secondary Lesions*

 Assessment

▲ Secondary lesions usually begin as a primary change or lesion in the skin (Figure 2–5):
- crust = dried serum or blood exudates
  - abrasion
  - ruptured blisters
- scar = connective tissue formed during the healing process that replaces skin damaged to the depth of the dermis
  - hypertrophied
  - atrophied
  - keloid
- fissure = linear crack in epidermis
  - chapping
  - cracked lips, as seen with dehydration
  - exposure
  - fever
- erosion = depressed, moist surface change affecting the epidermis
  - superficial scratch
  - syphilitic chancre
  - broken chickenpox vesicle

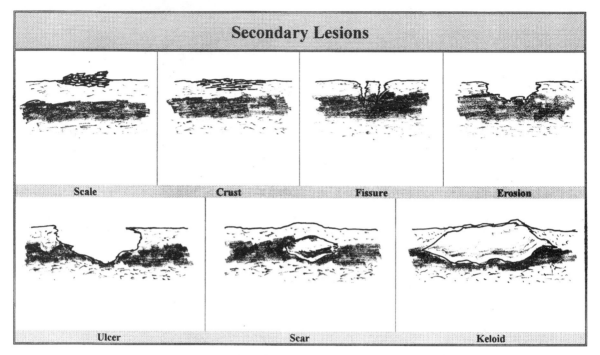

Figure 2–5. Secondary lesions.

- ulcer = necrotic hollowing of epidermis and dermis
  - decubiti
- scale = a flake of dead epithelium
  - psoriasis
  - seborrheic dermatitis
  - exfoliative dermatitis
- keloid = overproduction of scar tissue that appears raised, red, and smooth
  - high incidence of occurrence in African Americans

 Vascular Lesions

 Assessment

▲ Indicate trauma or systemic problems such as:
- clotting disorders
- leukemia
- infectious processes

▲ Ecchymoses = discoloration; various shades of red; yellow as time since onset increases; variable size
  • trauma
  • septicemia
  • hepatic dysfunction
  • bleeding disorders
▲ Hematoma = reddish purple or skin-toned, elevated, variable in size. Results from the collection of extravasated blood contained in the tissues of the skin
  • trauma
  • incomplete hemostasis after invasive procedure/surgery
▲ Petechiae = reddish-purple spots <0.5 cm, result from capillary bleeding, do not blanch
  • leukemia
  • inadequate or defective platelets
  • bacterial meningitis
▲ Purpura = reddish-purple spots >0.5 cm, do not blanch
  • thrombocytopenic purpura
  • intravascular defects
  • infection
▲ Spider angioma = bright-red center with radiating lines, blanches, usually found on face, neck, shoulders, upper chest
  • liver dysfunction
  • vitamin B deficiency
  • pregnancy
▲ Cherry angioma = bright-red, round lesions that may brown with age
  • nonpathologic
  • occurs with normal aging process
▲ Telangiectasia = dilation of capillaries and thinning of vascular walls that appear as bluish lines on the face and/or thighs
  • alcoholism
  • polycythemia
  • disorders with bleeding tendency
▲ Venous star = bluish areas that will not blanch and usually occur on legs or chest
  • increased pressure on superficial veins
  • venous distention

▶ *Contagious Rashes*

▲ Represents a risk of spreading infection to other individuals in the ED
▲ It is important for the triage nurse to be able to identify these rashes, and *appropriately isolate the patient directly from triage.*

 Assessment

Table 2–23 lists potentially contagious rashes.

TABLE 2–23 • Potentially Contagious Rashes

Problem	Rash Characteristics	Associated Signs and Symptoms
Measles	Generalized, papular, red blotchy rash	Koplik's spots in the mouth, runny nose, light sensitivity, fever, pruritus, cough
Chickenpox (varicella)	Vesicular, with crusting lesions in various stages; generalized Rash lesions are maculopapular for a few hours, vesicular for 3–4 days, and then leave a scab	Runny nose, fever, cough, pruritus
Impetigo	Vesicular, with crusting over erythematous base; localized initially, then spreading	
Scabies	Papules, vesicles, or linear rash, often between fingers, on neck and on forearms, but may be atypical	Severe persistent pruritis

► SYNCOPE

 Assessment

A. Obtain triage assessment that includes:
1. History:
   - ▲ visual changes
   - ▲ altered mental status
   - ▲ recent infections
   - ▲ chemical dependency
   - ▲ recent exercise
   - ▲ diet changes
   - ▲ known trauma
   - ▲ facial numbness
   - ▲ chemical or environmental exposure
   - ▲ medications (prescription and OTC)
   - ▲ medical conditions:
     - • cardiac
     - • neurologic
     - • pregnancy
     - • endocrine
2. Associated signs and symptoms:
   - ▲ dizziness
   - ▲ pallor
   - ▲ palpitations
   - ▲ malaise
   - ▲ weakness
   - ▲ ataxia
   - ▲ unsteady gait
   - ▲ speech irregularities
   - ▲ visual changes
   - ▲ vomiting
   - ▲ sudden, severe headache
   - ▲ irregular heartbeat
   - ▲ positive orthostatic vital signs
   - ▲ pupillary response abnormality
   - ▲ unequal hand grasps
   - ▲ altered mentation
   - ▲ numbness of face, arm, leg

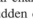 **Immediate Care If**

- ▲ Unstable vital signs
- ▲ Positive orthostatic vital signs
- ▲ Cardiac arrhythmias
- ▲ Blood loss
- ▲ Warning signs of stroke
  - • weakness or numbness
    - – face
    - – arm
    - – leg
    - – one side of body
  - • visual changes (especially unilateral)
    - – sudden dimness
    - – blurring
    - – decreased sight
  - • speech disturbances
    - – loss of language
    - – difficulty talking
    - – difficulty understanding conversation
    - – unexplained dizziness or vertigo
    - – decreased coordination
    - – sudden severe headache

Interventions

1. Provide for patient safety.
2. Maintain ABCs.

▶ TOXICOLOGY: BIOLOGICAL AND CHEMICAL EXPOSURE

Chemical and biological agents have been used in combat situations since the days of ancient Rome. In today's world, possible combat use by terrorists keeps biochemical warfare a very real threat to the health and well-being of our communities. It is essential for the triage nurse to be aware of these possibilities when assessing patients, since minutes may mean the difference between life and death for a patient exposed to a biological or chemical agent.

EDs need to be ready at any time for the threat of attack and the resulting influx of patients. To assist the country with understanding the day-to-day level of threat against our country, the government has devised a *Homeland Security Advisory System* (HSAS). This terror alert system will allow communities to understand where the threat is located and to what degree the risk is. The color-coded system in place is illustrated in Box 2–8.

Assessment

A. Obtain and record triage assessment
   1. Common signs and symptoms of **BIOLOGICAL** exposures (Table 2–24):
      ▲ headache
      ▲ runny nose

■ Box 2–8: HOMELAND SECURITY ADVISORY SYSTEM

Green (low condition) = A low risk of terrorist attack. The following may be applied:

• Refining and exercising preplanned protective measures
• Ensuring personnel receive training on HSAS, departmental, or agency-specific protective measures
• Regularly assessing facilities for vulnerabilities and taking measures to reduce the risks

Blue (guarded condition) = A general risk of terrorist attack. In addition to the above:

• The agencies should review and update their emergency response procedures

Yellow (elevated condition) = A significant risk of terrorist attack. In addition to the above:

• There is increased surveillance of critical locations
• Coordinating emergency plans with nearby jurisdictions
• The implementation of some emergency response plans are called for

Orange (high condition) = A significant high risk of terrorist attack. In addition to the above:

• The government will coordinate necessary security efforts with armed forces and/or law enforcement agencies
• Additional precautions are taken at public events
• Preparation to work at an alternate site or with a dispersed work force; and restrict access to essential personnel only

Red (severe condition) = A severe risk of terrorist attack. In addition to the above:

• Special teams of emergency response personnel may be required to be repositioned
• Public and governmental facilities will be closed
• Public transportation systems will be closely monitored, redirected, or constrained

TABLE 2-24 • Biological Agents

Agent and Incubation Period	Signs, Symptoms, Sequelae and Mode of Acquisition	Source	Vaccine Available	Contagious Between Humans	Treatment	Comments
ANTHRAX (INHALATION) *BACILLUS ANTHRACIS*						
7 days post-exposure	• Resembles a common cold (fever, cough, malaise), which progresses to severe dyspnea, diaphoresis, stridor, cyanosis, and shock • Chest x-ray shows a mediastinal widening • Gram-positive bacilli seen on blood smear and culture • Hemorrhagic mediastinitis, thoracic lymphadenitis, and/or meningitis • Inhalation of spores from contaminated animal products	• Infected animal tissue • Spores can live in the soil for years • Biological warfare agent	• Yes—approved for ages 18–65 years • 3 injections given 2 weeks apart, followed by 3 more injections at 6, 12, and 18 months	Extremely unlikely	• Early treatment is essential • Penicillin • Doxycycline • Fluoroquinolones (Cipro) • Special considerations for treatment of children, elderly, and pregnant women	• 90%–100% of cases are fatal
ANTHRAX (CUTANEOUS) *BACILLUS ANTHRACIS*						
7 days post-exposure	• Spores enter the skin • Infection more likely with a cut or abrasion on the skin • Infections begins with a raised, itchy bump that resembles a bug bite • Within 1–2 days, a vesicle develops, followed by a painless ulcer 1–3 cm in diameter, with a black necrotic center • Lymph glands in the adjacent area may swell	• Infected animal tissue, hair, fur, hides, leather • Spores can live in the soil for years • Biological warfare agent	• Yes—approved for ages 18–65 years • 3 injections given 2 weeks apart, followed by 3 more injections at 6, 12, and 18 months	Rare, but can occur	• Early treatment is essential • Penicillin • Doxycycline • Fluoroquinolones (Cipro) • Special considerations for treatment of children, elderly, and pregnant women	• Death rare if treated • 20% of untreated cases are fatal
ANTHRAX (INTESTINAL) *BACILLUS ANTHRACIS*						
7 days post-exposure	• Early symptoms: nausea, vomiting, malaise, anorexia, fever, acute inflammation of the GI tract • Advanced symptoms: abdominal pain, vomiting blood, severe diarrhea	• Infected animal tissue • Spores can live in the soil for years • Biological warfare agent	• Yes—approved for ages 18–65 years	Extremely unlikely	• Early treatment is essential • Penicillin • Doxycycline • Fluoroquinolones (Cipro)	• 25%–75% of cases are fatal

(continued)

TABLE 2-24 • Biological Agents (Continued)

Agent and Incubation Period	Signs, Symptoms, Sequelae and Mode of Acquisition	Source	Vaccine Available	Contagious Between Humans	Treatment	Comments
ANTHRAX (INTESTINAL) BACILLUS ANTHRACIS (continued)						
	• Illness progresses rapidly • Eating undercooked contaminated food		• 3 injections given 2 weeks apart, followed by 3 more injections at 6, 12, and 18 months		• Special considerations for treatment of children, elderly, and pregnant women	
BOTULISM (FOODBORNE) CLOSTRIDIUM BOTULINUM						
Incubation depends on amount and rate of toxin absorption; 2 hours–8 days	• Early symptoms: abdominal cramps, nausea, vomiting, diarrhea, difficulty seeing, speaking, swallowing • Double or blurred vision, drooping eyelids, slurred speech, dry mouth • Progresses to an acute, afebrile, symmetric, descending flaccid paralysis with multiple cranial nerve palsies, coma • The most poisonous substance known, a major bioweapon threat due to its extreme potency, lethality, ease of production, transport, and misuse	• Contaminated food from restaurants or home-canned sources • Bacteria commonly found in the soil	• Botulinum toxoid is available, but supplies are scarce and mass outbreaks of disease are rare	No	• Antitoxin available from CDC; must be administered early in course of disease • Supportive care	• Presents public health emergency • Mortality rate = 8%
BOTULISM (INHALED) CLOSTRIDIUM BOTULINUM						
Incubation depends on amount and rate of toxin absorption; 12–80 hours	• Ptosis, diplopia, blurred vision, dysarthria, dysphonia, dysphagia • Progresses to an acute, afebrile, symmetric, descending flaccid paralysis with multiple cranial nerve palsies, coma	• Man-made aerosolized form of the infection, created for use in bioterrorism	• Botulinum toxoid is available, but supplies are scarce and mass outbreaks of disease are rare	No	• Supportive care	• As above

• The most poisonous substance known, a major bioweapon threat due to its extreme potency, lethality, ease of production, transport, and misuse						

BOTULISM (WOUND) *CLOSTRIDIUM BOTULINUM*

Incubation depends on amount and rate of toxin absorption	• Double or blurred vision, drooping eyelids, slurred speech, dry mouth • Progresses to an acute, afebrile, symmetric, descending flaccid paralysis with multiple cranial nerve palsies, coma • Will NOT penetrate intact skin	• Bacteria found in soil—in recent years, black-tar heroin from California is a prime source	• As above	No	• Antitoxin available from CDC; must be administered early in course of disease • Supportive care	• Infectious disease that would **NOT** result from bioterrorism

BOTULISM (INTESTINAL) *CLOSTRIDIUM BOTULINUM*

	• Lethargy, feed poorly, constipation, weak cry, and poor muscle tone • Occasionally susceptible patients may harbor *C. botulinum* in their intestinal tract (most often occurs in infants)	• Bacteria commonly found in the soil	• As above	No	• Supportive care • Antitoxin is not routinely given for infant botulism	• Infectious disease that would **NOT** result from bioterrorism

BRUCELLOSIS (FOODBORNE) *BRUCELLA SPECIES*

Incubation is variable	• Flulike symptoms, such as fever, sweats, headache, back pain, and physical weakness • In severe cases, the patient may develop hepatitis, arthritis, spondylitis, anemia, leukopenia, thrombocytopenia, meningitis, uveitis, optic neuritis, papilledema, and endocarditis • Chronic symptoms may include recurrent fevers, joint pain, and fatigue	• Ingesting contaminated milk, dairy, or animal products • High risk in unpasteurized milk, ice cream, and cheeses	None available for humans	• Extremely rare, although may possibly be transmitted through breast milk, sexual contact, or tissue transplantation	• Doxycycline and rifampin used in combination for 6 weeks • Recovery takes a few weeks to several months	Mortality rate = <2%

TABLE 2–24 • Biological Agents (Continued)

Agent and Incubation Period	Signs, Symptoms, Sequelae and Mode of Acquisition	Source	Vaccine Available	Contagious Between Humans	Treatment	Comments
BRUCELLOSIS (INHALED) BRUCELLA SPECIES	As above	• Inhaling aerosolized *Brucella*	None available for humans	As above	As above	As above
BRUCELLOSIS (WOUND) BRUCELLA SPECIES	As above	• Transmitted via skin abrasions while handling infected animals	None available for humans	As above	As above	As above
PNEUMONIC PLAGUE YERSINIA PESTIS 1–6 days postexposure	• Early signs are fever, headache, weakness, dyspnea, and productive cough (bloody or watery sputum) • May see nausea, vomiting, abdominal pain, or diarrhea • Acutely swollen and painful lymph nodes appear on the 2nd day of the infection, and the overlying skin is erythematous • Pneumonia progresses over 2–4 days, followed by septic shock and death	• Bacteria carried by rodents and their fleas • Bioweapon usage would occur after aerosolization of the bacteria	None at this time; however, research is underway	Occurs through respiratory droplets during face-to-face contact	• Early treatment is important • Streptomycin • Tetracycline • Chloramphenicol • Doxycycline • Special considerations for treatment of children, elderly, and pregnant women • Respiratory isolation precautions: prophylactic antibiotic for close contacts of patient	• Death can occur in as little as 2–4 days
SMALLPOX (VARIOLA VIRUS) 7–17 days postexposure	• Initial symptoms are high fever, fatigue, head and back aches	• Infected saliva droplets	• U.S. has an emergency supply available (has not been routinely used since 1972)	• Occurs through respiratory droplets during face-to-face contact	• No proven treatment although research for antivirals continue	• Mortality rate = 30%

- 2–3 days later, a rash appears in the mouth, on the face, arms, and legs. The rash begins as flat red lesions that evolve at the same rate—after a day or 2, the lesions become pus filled and begin to crust early in the 2nd week. Scabs fall off after 3–4 weeks.
- Patients with smallpox are most infectious during the first week of illness, although are contagious until all skin scabs are healed
- In people exposed to smallpox, the vaccine can be given within 4 days to lessen or prevent the illness

- Can also be transmitted by contaminated clothing or bedding

- Supportive care should include IV fluids, antipyretics, and antibiotics for secondary infections
- Patients admitted to the hospital should be placed in negative pressure rooms; staff should use standard precautions to protect against spread of the disease

TULAREMIA *FRANCISELLA TURARENSIS*

1–14 days post-exposure

- Initial symptoms are fever, pharyngitis, headache, body aches, and upper respiratory illness, rapidly progressing to bronchitis, pneumonia, pleuropneumonitis, bacteremia
- May see nausea, weight loss, malaise with continued illness
- Inhalation would have the greatest adverse public health consequences—release in a densely populated area would result in an abrupt onset of a sick population (slower progression than anthrax or plague)

- Contaminated arthropods, soil, animals, water, and vegetation
- Humans become infected by direct contact, ingestion, or inhaled infective aerosols

Vaccine available, not fully approved for general use

No

- Individual treatment drugs of choice:
  - streptomycin
  - gentamycin
- Mass casualty treatment drugs of choice:
  - doxycycline
  - ciprofloxacin

<2% mortality rate

(continued)

TABLE 2–24 • Biological Agents (Continued)

Agent and Incubation Period	Signs, Symptoms, Sequelae and Mode of Acquisition	Source	Vaccine Available	Contagious Between Humans	Treatment	Comments
TULAREMIA *FRANCISELLA TURARENSIS* (continued)	• This is a dangerous bioweapon due to its extreme infectivity, ease of dissemination, and substantial capacity to cause illness and death				• Special considerations for children, pregnant woman, and those with immuno-suppression	
VIRAL HEMORRHAGIC FEVERS (VHF)	• VHF is a term used to describe a severe multisystem syndrome in which the overall vascular system is damaged • Initially, fever, fatigue, dizziness, muscle aches, weakness, and extreme fatigue are seen in the patient • Severe infections will produce bleeding under the skin (petechiae), internal bleeding, or bleeding from body orifices • These patients will progress to shock, nervous system malfunction, coma, delirium, seizures, and/or renal failure • VHF refers to a group of illnesses caused by several families of viruses: • Arenaviruses (Argentine, Bolivian, Lassa) • Bunyaviruses (Rift Valley, Hantavirus) • Filoviruses (Ebola, Marburg) • Flaviviruses (Tickborne, Kyasanur Forest)	• Most VHFs are insect or animal borne • The vector for Ebola and Marburg viruses are unknown • Humans become infected through contact with rodent's bodily fluids or when bitten by an arthropod	• Available only for yellow fever and Argentine hemorrhagic fever at this time • No vaccines exist for the other VHFs	• Humans may transmit some of these VHFs to other humans	• There are no treatments for most of the VHFs • Supportive care is given	• Mortality rate varies with each VHF—most are between 50%–90% mortality rate

Q FEVER *COXIELLA BURNETII*

2–3 weeks post-exposure	Symptoms	Transmission	Vaccine	Person-to-person	Treatment	Mortality
	• Sudden onset of high fever (104°–105°F), severe headache, malaise, myalgia, confusion, sore throat, chills, sweats, nonproductive cough, nausea, vomiting, diarrhea, abdominal pain, chest pain • Fever lasts for 1–2 weeks • 30%–50% of patients develop pneumonia • This agent is highly infectious and resistant to heat, drying, and most disinfectants. It easily becomes airborne and is inhaled by humans, and therefore is at risk of abuse by bioterrorists. • Chronic Q fever occurs when infection persists for >6 months—these patients are prone to endocarditis	• Infected milk, urine, feces, amniotic fluid of animals • Humans are infected by inhaling dried, contaminated particles • Ingestion of contaminated milk may produce illness	Yes, although not commercially available in the U.S.	Rare	Q fever: • Doxycycline—most efficient when started within first 3 days of illness Chronic Q fever: • Doxycycline with quinolones for at least 4 years or • Doxycycline with hydrochloroquine for 1.5–3 years	Q fever: <2% mortality rate Chronic Q fever: 65% mortality rate

(Arnon, 2001; CDC, 2001; Inglesby, 2000; CDC, 1997; Henderson, 1999; Dennis, 2001)
(Reprinted with permission from www.RN.CEUS.COM)

- ▲ blurred vision
- ▲ slurred speech
- ▲ difficulty swallowing or dry mouth
- ▲ cough
- ▲ difficulty breathing
- ▲ swollen lymph glands
- ▲ muscle or joint pain
- ▲ weight loss
- ▲ fever
- ▲ nausea/vomiting/diarrhea
- ▲ abdominal pain
- ▲ raised red rash
- ▲ petechiae
- ▲ bleeding from body orifices

2. Common signs and symptoms of **CHEMICAL** exposures (Table 2–25):
- ▲ runny nose
- ▲ drooling
- ▲ blurred vision
- ▲ tearing of eyes
- ▲ eyelid swelling
- ▲ headache
- ▲ chest tightness
- ▲ difficulty breathing
- ▲ nausea/vomiting/diarrhea
- ▲ incontinence of urine or stool
- ▲ muscle cramps or twitching
- ▲ rash
- ▲ burns to the skin, eyes, nares, airway
- ▲ confusion
- ▲ convulsions
- ▲ paralysis
- ▲ coma

B. Identify known exposure or the possibility of biochemical exposure by:

1. Obtaining specific detailed history from patient, including:
- ▲ recent travel history
- ▲ recent activity history (social situations)
- ▲ work environment
- ▲ living situation
- ▲ dietary history
- ▲ any unusual letters or packages handled recently

2. Identify possible community considerations:
- ▲ Does the patient know anyone else with similar symptoms?
- ▲ Has the health care provider seen any unusual clusters of symptoms, illnesses, or diseases?

3. Work closely with hospital team and Department of Health in identification of suspicious events that may indicate a possible bioterrorist act:
- ▲ outbreak of a large number of cases of acute flaccid paralysis with prominent bulbar palsies (botulism)

TABLE 2-25 • Chemical Agents

Agents and Descriptions	Onset of Symptoms Postexposure	Signs and Symptoms, Routes of Exposure	Action, Risks	Decontamination and Treatment
NERVE AGENTS				
Sarin Pure liquid is clear, colorless, tasteless; becomes brown with aging	• Immediately if inhaled, may be several hours if it touches the skin	• Runny nose, watery eyes, drooling, blurred vision, headache, excessive sweating, chest tightness, difficulty breathing, nausea, vomiting, loss of bowel/bladder control, muscle cramps, twitching, confusion, convulsions, paralysis, and coma • Can enter the body by inhalation, ingestion, through the eyes and skin	• Chemicals that attack the nervous system by binding with acetylcholinesterase, allowing acetylcholine to overstimulate the glands and voluntary muscles until they fail • Lethal—1 drop on the skin can cause death in less than 15 minutes	• **Skin:** Remove contaminated clothing (double-bag in plastic bags and seal) and wash skin with large amount of soap and water or 5% bleach. Rinse well with water. • **Eyes:** Immediately flush eyes with water for 10-15 minutes—do NOT cover eyes with patches afterwards • **Ingestion:** Do NOT induce vomiting. If patient is alert and able to swallow, immediately administer activated charcoal. • **Vapor:** Remove outer clothing and place in sealed double bag. Care for exposed skin as above. • **Emergency treatment and antidotes:** Maintain airway, cardiac monitor, IVs, monitor vital signs. Follow ACLS protocols. Administer atropine (2 mg for adults, 0.05–.1 mg/kg for children) every 5–10 minutes until respiratory status stabilizes, antidote (2-PAM Cl), and diazepam for seizures (barbiturates and phenytoin are not effective).
VX Amber-colored, tasteless, odorless oily liquid	• Onset of symptoms vary based on route of exposure • VX absorbs very rapidly through the eyes • At least 100 times more toxic than Sarin with skin entry and twice as toxic by inhalation	• Runny nose, watery eyes, drooling, excessive sweating, chest tightness, dyspnea, pinpoint pupils, nausea, vomiting, abdominal cramps, incontinences of bowel or bladder, twitching, headache, confusion, coma, or seizures • Can enter the body by inhalation, ingestion, through the eyes and skin	• Kills by binding acetylcholinesterase. This causes constant stimulation of glands and voluntary muscles until ultimate fatigue and a cessation of breathing ability • Extremely lethal and persistent—can last for months in cold weather, evaporates 1,500 times slower than water	• **Skin:** Remove contaminated clothing and wash skin with large amounts of soap and water, 10% sodium carbonate, or 5% liquid household bleach. Rinse well with water. Administer antidote only if local sweating and muscular twitching is present. • **Eyes:** *Immediately* flush eyes with water for 10-15 minutes, then place respiratory protective mask. Use antidote only if more symptoms than just miosis occur. VX absorbs 100 times faster through the eyes than Sarin does. • **Ingestion:** Do NOT induce vomiting. • **Inhalation:** Use positive pressure full-face breathing mask. Do NOT perform mouth-to-mouth on a patient with VX exposure! Immediately administer nerve agent antidote.

(continued)

TABLE 2–25 • Chemical Agents (Continued)

Agents and Descriptions	Onset of Symptoms Postexposure	Signs and Symptoms, Routes of Exposure	Action, Risks	Decontamination and Treatment
VX (continued)		• Death can occur within 15 minutes of absorption of fatal dosage		• **Emergency treatment and antidotes:** Maintain airway, cardiac monitor, IVs, monitor vital signs. Follow ACLS protocols. Administer atropine (2 mg for adults, 0.05–.1 mg/kg for children) every 5–10 minutes until respiratory status stabilizes, antidote (2-PAM Cl), and diazepam for seizures (barbiturates and phenytoin are not effective).
GF (Cyclohexyl Sarin) Colorless and odorless liquid in pure form	• Depending on the dose, onset of symptoms occurs within minutes or hours • Rapid absorption through the eyes	• Runny nose, miosis, headache, dyspnea, chest tightness, cough, drooling, excessive sweating, copious sinus secretions, nausea, vomiting, abdominal cramps, diarrhea, incontinence of bowel and bladder, muscle twitching and weakness, confusion, apnea, coma, death • Can enter the body by inhalation, ingestion, through the eyes and skin	• Organophosphorus compound, a lethal cholinesterase inhibitor similar in action to Sarin	• **Skin:** Remove contaminated clothing and wash skin with large amounts of soap and water, 10% sodium carbonate, or 5% liquid household bleach. Rinse well with water. Administer antidote only if local sweating and muscular twitching is present. • **Eyes:** *Immediately* flush eyes with water for 10–15 minutes, then place respiratory protective mask. Only use antidote if more symptoms than just miosis occur. • **Ingestion:** Do NOT induce vomiting. Immediately administer nerve agent antidote. • **Inhalation:** Use positive-pressure full-face, self-contained breathing apparatus. For severe signs, immediately administer nerve agent antidote and oxygen. Do NOT perform mouth-to-mouth resuscitation if face is contaminated with GF. • **Emergency treatment and antidotes:** Maintain airway, cardiac monitor, IVs, monitor vital signs. Follow ACLS protocols. Administer atropine (2 mg for adults, 0.05–.1 mg/kg for children) every 5–10 minutes until respiratory status stabilizes, antidote (2-PAM CL), and diazepam for seizures (barbiturates and phenytoin are not effective).
PULMONARY AGENTS Nitrogen Oxide Red/brown gas or a yellow liquid with pungent odor	• The substance and vapor irritate the eyes,	• Cough, wheezing, sore throat, dizziness, headache, sweating, dyspnea,	• Causes lung edema • Exposure of high amounts can cause death	• **Skin:** Rinse with plenty of water, then remove contaminated clothing and rinse again. Refer for medical attention.

Agent	Symptoms	Health Effects	First Aid
skin, and respiratory tract • Effects may be delayed	vomiting, or redness at point of contact (eyes, skin) • Can enter the body by inhalation or ingestion		• **Eyes:** Flush eyes with water for 10–15 minutes (be sure to remove contact lenses), then refer for medical attention. • **Ingestion:** Rinse mouth with copious amounts of water. • **Inhalation:** Apply oxygen; place in sitting position. Seek medical evaluation.
Chlorine Green/yellow gas with pungent odor • Effects may be delayed	• Very corrosive effects • Tearing of the eyes, headache, sore throat, cough, dyspnea, burning sensation, lung edema, frostbite, burns to the skin, nausea, eye pain, blurred vision • Enters the body by inhalation	• Corrosive effects to lungs, skin, and eyes • Chronic exposure results in erosion of the teeth, chronic bronchitis • Overexposure can cause death	• **Skin:** Remove contaminated clothing, then rinse skin with plenty of water or a shower. Seek medical help for burns. • **Eyes:** Flush eyes with water for 10–15 minutes (be sure to remove contact lenses), then refer for medical attention. • **Inhalation:** Apply oxygen; place in sitting position. May need artificial ventilation. Seek medical evaluation.
Sulphur Dioxide Colorless gas or compressed liquefied gas with pungent odor • Inhalation symptoms may be delayed • Contact with skin can cause immediate frostbite	• Frostbite to the skin, eye pain with redness and severe burns, sore throat, cough, dyspnea, lung edema, reflex spasm of the larynx, respiratory arrest, death • Enters the body by inhalation	• Strong irritant to the eyes and respiratory tract • Repeated or prolonged exposure can cause asthma	• **Skin:** Remove contaminated clothing, then rinse with plenty of water. Do NOT remove clean clothing. Seek medical help for frostbite. • **Eyes:** Flush eyes with water for 10–15 minutes (be sure to remove contact lenses), then refer for medical attention. • **Inhalation:** Apply oxygen; place in sitting position. May need artificial ventilation. Seek medical evaluation.
Phosgene Colorless gas or colorless to yellow compressed	• Frostbite to the skin, eye pain with redness and severe burns, blurred	• Corrosive to skin, respiratory tract, and eyes	• **Skin:** Remove contaminated clothing, then rinse with plenty of water. Do NOT remove clean clothing. Seek medical help for frostbite.

(continued)

TABLE 2–25 • Chemical Agents (Continued)

Agents and Descriptions	Onset of Symptoms Postexposure	Signs and Symptoms, Routes of Exposure	Action, Risks	Decontamination and Treatment
PULMONARY AGENTS (continued)				
liquefied gas with characteristic odor	• Contact with skin can cause immediate frostbite	vision, sore throat, cough, dyspnea, lung edema, death • Enters the body by inhalation	• Long-term exposure may result in lung fibrosis	• **Eyes:** Flush eyes with water for 10–15 minutes (be sure to remove contact lenses), then refer for medical attention. • **Inhalation:** Apply oxygen; place in sitting position. May need artificial ventilation. Seek medical evaluation.
Titanium Tetrachloride Colorless to light yellow liquid with pungent odor	• Symptoms may be delayed	• Red painful eyes with burns, skin blisters, cough, dyspnea, chest tightness, abdominal pain, shock, coma • Enters the body by inhalation or ingestion.	• Corrosive to skin, eyes, respiratory and GI tracts. • Can cause permanent eye damage • Long-term exposure may result in lung impairment.	• **Skin:** Remove contaminated clothing, rinse with plenty of water, then wash with soap and water. • **Eyes:** Flush eyes with water for 10–15 minutes (be sure to remove contact lenses), then refer for medical attention. • **Ingestion:** Rinse mouth. Do NOT induce vomiting. Seek medical attention immediately. • **Inhalation:** Apply oxygen; place in sitting position. May need artificial ventilation. Seek medical evaluation.
BLISTER AGENTS **Lewisite** Amber to dark brown liquid with a strong, penetrating, geranium odor. The pure compound is a colorless, odorless, oily liquid.	• Immediate symptoms with eye exposure, inhalation, or ingestion • Skin contact produces symptoms within 30 minutes	• Eyelid swelling, severe eye pain, iritis, copious sinus drainage, violent sneezing, cough, frothing mucus, lung edema, large skin blisters and burns, diarrhea, hypothermia, hypotension • Severe irritation and lung edema. Can cause systemic poisoning, hemoconcentration, shock, and death	• Causes blindness *within 1 minute* of exposure • Nonfatal hemolysis results in anemia • Metabolites excreted by liver cause focal necrosis of liver, biliary passages, and intestine • Long-term exposure can cause chronic lung impairment and cancer	• **Skin:** Immediately wash skin and clothes with 5% sodium hypochlorite or household bleach within 1 minute of exposure, then cut and remove contaminated cloth. Rewash skin again with 5% liquid household bleach. Then wash contaminated skin a 3rd time with soap and water. • **Eyes:** Immediately flush eyes with water for 10–15 minutes. • **Ingestion:** Rinse mouth. Do NOT induce vomiting. Give patient milk to drink. • **Inhalation:** Apply oxygen, place in sitting position. May need artificial ventilation. Do NOT perform mouth-to-mouth if facial contamination has occurred.

Agent		Effects	Treatment
	• Can enter the body by inhalation, ingestion, through the eyes and skin		
Mustard Gas Pure liquid is colorless and odorless. Agent-grade material is yellow, brown, or black with a sweet-type odor of garlic or horseradish.	• Rapid penetration of moist mucous membranes and skin • Delayed severe symptoms of the respiratory tract	• Severe tearing and pain of eyes with possible blindness, sneezing, coughing, anorexia, diarrhea, fever, skin blisters • Can enter the body by inhalation, ingestion, through the eyes and skin. Tender skin, mucous membranes, and perspiration-covered skin is more vulnerable	• Causes delayed serve damage to the respiratory tract and cytotoxic action on hematopoietic tissues • Lethal doses are carcinogens and teratogenics • Distilled mustard is nearly pure, while mustard gas is only 70%–80% pure

• **Skin:** Immediately wash skin and clothes with 5% sodium hypochlorite or household bleach within 1 minute of exposure, then cut and remove contaminated cloth. Flush skin again with 5% sodium hypochlorite solution, then wash contaminated skin a 3rd time with soap and water.

• **Eyes:** Immediately flush eyes with water for 10–15 minutes. Do not cover with bandages. Use dark goggles or glasses.

• **Ingestion:** Do NOT induce vomiting. Give patient milk to drink.

• **Inhalation:** Apply oxygen; place in sitting position. May need artificial ventilation. Do NOT perform mouth-to-mouth if facial contamination has occurred.

BLOOD AGENTS:

Agent		Effects	Treatment
Arsine Colorless compressed liquefied gas with a characteristic odor	• Immediate to delayed symptoms, depending on exposure	• Causes immediate frostbite when contact made with eyes or skin • Headache, confusion, dizziness, nausea, vomiting, abdominal pain, dyspnea, lung edema, kidney failure, damage to blood cells, death • Enters the body by inhalation	• Chronic exposure is carcinogenic to humans

• **Skin:** Remove contaminated clothing, then rinse with plenty of water. Do NOT remove clean clothing. Seek medical help for frostbite.

• **Eyes:** Flush eyes with water for 10–15 minutes followed by an immediate eye exam.

• **Inhalation:** Apply oxygen; place in sitting position. May need artificial ventilation.

(continued)

TABLE 2–25 • Chemical Agents (Continued)

Agents and Descriptions	Onset of Symptoms Postexposure	Signs and Symptoms, Routes of Exposure	Action, Risks	Decontamination and Treatment
Cyanogen Chloride Colorless compressed liquefied gas with a pungent odor	• Effects of exposure may be delayed	• Causes immediate frostbite with contact to eyes/skin • Sore throat, severe tearing, confusion, drowsiness, unconsciousness, nausea, vomiting, lung edema • Enters the body by inhalation or absorbed through the skin	• Overexposure results in death	• **Skin:** Remove contaminated clothing, then rinse with plenty of water. Do NOT remove clean clothing. Seek medical help for frostbite. • **Eyes:** Flush eyes with water for 10–15 minutes followed by an immediate eye exam. • **Inhalation:** Apply oxygen; place in sitting position. May need artificial ventilation.
Hydrogen Chloride Colorless compressed liquefied gas with a pungent odor	• Highly corrosive symptoms may begin immediately or be delayed	• Corrosive, deep, severe burns to eyes and skin • Sore throat, blurred vision, coughing, dyspnea, lung edema, burning sensation • Enters the body through inhalation	• Long-term exposure may cause erosion to the teeth or chronic bronchitis	• **Skin:** Remove contaminated clothing, then rinse with plenty of water. Seek treatment for burns. • **Eyes:** Flush eyes with water for 10–15 minutes followed by an immediate eye exam. • **Inhalation:** Apply oxygen; place in sitting position. May need artificial ventilation.
Hydrogen Cyanide Colorless gas or liquid with a characteristic odor	• Highly irritating—symptoms may be immediate or delayed	• Headache, confusion, drowsiness, dyspnea, loss of consciousness, nausea, skin and eye redness and pain, burning sensation • Enters the body through inhalation, ingestion, eye and skin absorption • Easily absorbed as a vapor or through the skin or eyes	• May injure central nervous, respiratory, and circulatory systems • Exposure may cause death	• **Skin:** Flush skin with plenty of water or take a shower. Wear gloves when administering first aid. • **Eyes:** Immediately flush eyes with water for 10–15 minutes, then seek eye exam. • **Ingestion:** Rinse mouth immediately. Do NOT induce vomiting. • **Inhalation:** Apply oxygen; place in sitting position. May need artificial ventilation. Avoid mouth-to-mouth resuscitation.

(CDC, 2001; CDC, 2002)

▲ large numbers of patients with a similar disease, syndrome, or cluster of symptoms
▲ outbreak of botulism with a common geographic factor among cases (e.g., airport, work location) but without a common dietary exposure (e.g., features suggestive of an aerosol attack)
▲ multiple simultaneous outbreaks of similar illnesses with no common source
▲ an increase in unexplained diseases or death with or without a common disease or syndrome
▲ unusual illness in a population
  • e.g., renal disease (could be caused by exposure to mercury)
▲ patients failing to respond to usual therapies or treatment for common illnesses
▲ single case of unusual disease
  • smallpox
  • VHF
  • anthrax
▲ illnesses occurring outside of season, normal location, or normal age group such as:
  • tularemia in a nonendemic area, or influenza in the summer
  • chickenpox in adult
▲ unexplainable sudden increase in cases of a normally seen disease
▲ atypical disease transmission may signal the possibility of sabotage of food source
▲ many ill patients seeking similar treatment for similar symptoms at the same time

Interventions

If the suspicion of possible exposure exists, or there is a known exposure, the patient(s) must be immediately brought into the ED for care. Refer to hospital policy for events to occur, and refer to Tables 2–26 through 2–28 for further information.

TABLE 2-26 • Prehospital Triage of Mass Casualty Patients: Nerve Agents

Triage Priority	Priority Description	Current State	Clinical Signs
IMMEDIATE	• Patients who require lifesaving care within a short period of time • Emergency care must be available and of short duration • This care may include emergency measures that are performed within a few minutes time, such as intubation or antidote administration	• Unconscious • Talking but unable to walk • Moderate to severe effects of two or more organs or systems (e.g., respiratory, GI, etc.)	• Seizing or postictal • Severe respiratory distress • Cardiac arrest (recovered)
DELAYED	• Patients with severe injuries in need of major surgery, require hospitalization, or other care—but a delay in care will not adversely affect the outcome of this patient, e.g., internal stabilization of a fracture	• Recovering from recent exposure or antidote administration	• Diminished secretions • Improving or stable respiratory status
MINIMAL	• Patients who have minor injuries who can be helped by nonmedical personnel and who won't require hospitalization	• Walking and talking	• Miosis • Rhinorrhea • Mild to moderate dyspnea
EXPECTANT	• Patients with severe life-threatening injuries who probably would not survive even with the best of medical attention • Patients with injuries that require attention from many medical personnel but have a low chance of survival do not justify the use of limited medical resources • As this mass casualty event changes, these patients may be retriaged once additional medical resources become available	• Unconscious	• Cardiac arrest • Respiratory arrest

(CDC, 2001; ATSDR, 2001)

TABLE 2-27 • Prehospital Antidote Management: When Military Mark I Kits Are Not Available

Patient Age	Mild Symptoms	Severe Symptoms
	(Localized sweating; difficulty breathing; nausea, vomiting, diarrhea; muscle fasciculations, weakness)	(Apnea, seizures, flaccid paralysis, unconsciousness)
Infant: <2 years old	Atropine: 0.05 mg/kg IM 2-PAM Cl: 15 mg/kg IM	Atropine: 0.1 mg/kg IM 2-PAM Cl: 25 mg/kg IM
Children: 2–10 years old	Atropine: 1 mg IM 2-PAM Cl: 15 mg/kg IM	Atropine: 2 mg IM 2-PAM Cl: 25 mg/kg IM
Adolescent: >10 years old	Atropine: 2 mg IM 2-PAM Cl: 15 mg/kg IM	Atropine: 4 mg IM 2-PAM Cl: 25 mg/kg IM
Adult	Atropine: 2–4 mg IM 2-PAM Cl: 600 mg IM	Atropine: 6 mg IM 2-PAM Cl: 1800 mg IM
Frail elderly	Atropine: 1 mg IM 2-PAM Cl: 10 mg/kg IM	Atropine: 2–4 mg IM 2-PAM Cl: 25 mg/kg IM

Alert:
• 2-PAM Cl solution needs to be reconstituted from the vial containing 1 g of desiccated 2-PAM Cl with 3 mL of saline, 5% distilled water, or sterile water into the vial and shake well. Resulting solution is 3.3 mL of 300 mg/mL.
• Assisted ventilation should be started after the administration of the antidote for severe cases of exposure.
• Repeat the atropine every 5–10 minutes until secretions have diminished and breathing has returned to baseline.

(CDC, 2001; ATSDR, 2001)

TABLE 2-28 • Emergency Department Antidote Management

Patient Age	Mild Symptoms	Severe Symptoms
	(Localized sweating; difficulty breathing; nausea, vomiting, diarrhea; muscle fasciculations, weakness)	(Apnea, seizures, flaccid paralysis, unconsciousness)
Infant: <2 years old	Atropine: 0.05 mg/kg IM or 0.02 mg/kg IV 2-PAM Cl: 15 mg/kg IV slowly	Atropine: 0.1 mg/kg IM or 0.02 mg/kg IV 2-PAM Cl: 15 mg/kg IV slowly
Children: 2–10 years old	Atropine: 1 mg IM 2-PAM Cl: 15 mg/kg IV slowly	Atropine: 2 mg IM 2-PAM Cl: 15 mg/kg IV slowly
Adolescent: >10 years old	Atropine: 2 mg IM 2-PAM Cl: 15 mg/kg IV slowly	Atropine: 4 mg IM 2-PAM Cl: 15 mg/kg IV slowly
Adult	Atropine: 2–4 mg IM 2-PAM Cl: 15 mg/kg (1 g) IV slowly	Atropine: 6 mg IM 2-PAM Cl: 15 mg/kg (1 g) IV slowly
Frail elderly	Atropine: 1 mg IM 2-PAM Cl: 5–10 mg/kg IV slowly	Atropine: 2 mg IM 2-PAM Cl: 5–10 mg/kg IV slowly

Alert:
• 2-PAM Cl solution may need to be reconstituted from the vial containing 1 gram of desiccated 2-PAM Cl with 3 mL of saline, 5% distilled water, or sterile water into the vial and shake well. Resulting solution is 3.3 mL of 300 mg/mL.
• Use phentolamine for hypertension induced by 2-PAM Cl (5 mg IV for adults, 1 mg IV for children).
• Use diazepam for seizure control (0.2–0.5 mg IV for <5 years old; 1 mg IV for children >5 years old; 5 mg IV for adults).
• Repeat atropine every 5–10 minutes until secretions have diminished and dyspnea relieved (for infants, use 2 mg IM or 1 mg IV).

(CDC, 2001; ATSDR, 2001)

TRAUMA, MULTIPLE (ADULT)

Report of incoming trauma patients often comes in the form of the mnemonic MIVT. The ED staff should understand this form to be prepared for their trauma patient. This mnemonic stands for:

M = **M**echanism of injury
I = **I**njuries sustained
V = **V**ital signs
T = **T**reatment before arrival

Any victim of trauma cared for in your department will be evaluated and treated according to your hospital's ED trauma protocol. The following is a brief outline of the sequence of events that will occur. The ED team will *need to adjust* the protocol to meet the *individual needs* of each trauma victim.

 Assessment and Interventions

A. When notification of an incoming trauma victim is received, the ED charge/triage nurse must immediately:
  1. Communicate to appropriate personnel
    ▲ ED physician
    ▲ nursing supervisor
    ▲ ED nursing and ancillary staff
    ▲ ancillary services such as:
      • operating room
      • registration
      • laboratory
      • trauma or code team, as needed
      • respiratory therapy
      • radiology
      • ECG
      • social worker (for family members)
  2. Assign staff who will care for other ED patients.
  3. Prepare trauma room, verify available setup of:
    ▲ oxygen (non-rebreather mask and ambu-bag ready)
    ▲ suction (prepare two setups)
    ▲ cardiac monitor in "on" position
    ▲ position BP machine, oximeter, and thermometer at bedside
    ▲ IV solutions, tubing, supplies
    ▲ open appropriate cart if need indicates
    ▲ critical care flow sheet for documentation
    ▲ universal precaution protection equipment
    ▲ assign staff roles in trauma care
      • documentation
      • IV
      • medications

- Foley catheter
- other duties, as applicable

B. When patient arrives, the ED team will:
1. Obtain brief report from Emergency Medical Service (EMS) crew.
2. Assist with patient transfer from EMS stretcher onto trauma stretcher *while maintaining c-spine and airway precautions.*
C. Perform primary survey and intervene immediately as necessary:
1. Airway with c-spine control
    ▲ clear and open airway:
      - administer oxygen by mask
    ▲ partially or potentially obstructed airway:
      - clear obstruction if possible, carefully observe, administer oxygen
    ▲ obstructed airway:
      - prepare for intubation or crichothyrotomy
2. Breathing:
    ▲ assess rate, depth, regularity, and ease of respiratory effort
    ▲ assess for use of accessory and abdominal muscles
    ▲ assess for chest wall integrity and symmetry of expansion
    ▲ assess for decreased level of consciousness
    ▲ assess for cyanosis
3. Circulation:
    ▲ assess pulse quality, location and rate
      - if *radial* pulse is present, systolic BP is at least 80 mmHg
      - if *femoral* pulse is present, systolic BP is at least 70 mmHg
      - if *carotid* pulse is present, systolic BP is at least 60 mmHg
    ▲ place patient on cardiac monitor, run a strip
    ▲ assess capillary refill (normal is 1–2 sec)
    ▲ assess skin color
    ▲ note obvious sources of bleeding
    ▲ assess level of consciousness
    ▲ apply BP cuff (manual or machine)
    ▲ apply oximetry probe, correlate pulse to verify $SAO_2\%$ reading
    ▲ insert IVs as indicated, usually two large-bore catheters (14–18 gauge)
    ▲ obtain blood samples
4. Disability:
    ▲ assess level of consciousness
    ▲ obtain subjective data including:
      - mechanism of injury (Table 2–29; Box 2–9)
      - patient complaints
      - areas of pain, numbness, tingling, and ability to move
      - treatment at accident scene and before arrival
      - allergies
      - current medications, including anticoagulants, ETOH, or use of illegal drugs
    ▲ last tetanus immunization
      - past medical and surgical history
      - any family, friends, or clergy the patient wants called

TABLE 2–29 • Mechanisms of Injury from Trauma: Adult

Trauma	Associated Injuries
Pedestrian struck by car adult point of impact is usually knee/hip	Fractures of the femur, tibia, and fibula on side of impact Fractured pelvis Contralateral ligament damage to knee

Pedestrian struck by car
  short adult/child point of impact involves
  chest and or head
	Contralateral skull fracture
	Chest injury with rib and/or sternal fracture
	May be thrown, resulting in head/back injury
	Shoulder dislocation and/or scapular fracture
	Patellar and lower femur fracture

Pedestrian dragged under a vehicle	Pelvic fracture
Unrestrained: front-seat passenger front impact	Posterior dislocation of acetabulum Fractures of femurs and/or patellas
Unrestrained: driver front impact	Head injury, c-spine injury, pelvic fracture Flail chest, fractured sternum Aortic or tracheal tears Pulmonary/cardiac contusion Ruptured or lacerated liver or spleen Femur and/or patellar fracture, hip dislocation
Unrestrained: driver or passenger side impact	Chest: flail, fractured sternum, pulmonary/cardiac contusion Fractures of clavicle, acetabulum, pelvis Lateral neck strain or injury Driver: ruptured spleen Passenger: ruptured liver
Passenger: without headrest restraint rear impact	Hyperextension of neck resulting in high c-spine or vertebral fracture or ruptured disk, causing intradural hemorrhage, edema, cord compression
Rotational force from spinning car	Combination of frontal and side impact-induced injuries
Rollover of vehicle	Multitude of external and internal injuries
Ejection from vehicle	Injuries at point of impact
Restrained: driver or passenger	Compression of soft tissue organs, c-spine injuries, rib and sternal fractures, cardiac contusions, ruptured diaphragm Lap belt only: head, neck, facial, and chest injuries Shoulder strap only: severe neck injury, decapitation Air bag deployed: facial injuries, abrasions/burns of arms
Fall landing on feet	Compression fractures of lumbosacral spine Fractures of calcaneus
Fall landing on buttocks	Compression fracture of lumbar vertebrae Pelvic fracture Coccyx fracture
Diving head first	Forceful cervical spine compression resulting in fracture, dislocation, and/or vertebral bone fragments displaced into spinal canal

TABLE 2-29 • Mechanisms of Injury from Trauma: Adult (Continued)

Trauma	Associated Injuries

Blunt head trauma
   person's moving head strikes a
   stationary object
	Coup/contracoup injury
	Depressed skull fracture
	Cerebral hematoma, contusions, or laceration

Blunt chest trauma moving object strikes a person's chest	Pulmonary contusion Hemothorax Rib fractures

Crush injury to chest	Traumatic asphyxia:
	   crushing trauma to chest forces blood from heart via the superior
	   vena cava to veins of the head, neck, and upper chest, causing:
	      subconjunctival and retinal hemorrhage
	      conjunctival edema
	      characteristic deep-violet skin color

■ Box 2-9: TRIAGE QUESTIONS FOR PATIENTS INVOLVED IN A MOTOR VEHICLE ACCIDENT

- When did the accident occur?
  - day
  - time
- Where did it occur?
  - highway
  - country road
  - city street
  - off-road
  - speedway
- Was the patient wearing a seat belt?
  - what type? (lap, shoulder, etc.)
  - effectiveness during the accident?
- What speed was the patient's car traveling?
  - approximate speed of other vehicles involved in accident
  - approximate speed of patient's vehicle
- Where was the patient sitting in the car?
  - driver
  - front-seat passenger
  - back-seat passenger
  - box of the truck
- What kind of vehicle was the patient in?
  - What damage was done to the vehicle?
- Did the airbag deploy?
- Did the patient lose consciousness?
  - for how long?

(continued)

■ Box 2-9: **TRIAGE QUESTIONS FOR PATIENTS INVOLVED IN A MOTOR VEHICLE ACCIDENT (Continued)**

- What is the last thing the patient remembers *before* the accident?
- What is the first thing the patient remembers *after* the accident?
- How was the patient injured in the car?
  - flying objects within the car?
  - car crushed by other vehicle, tree, pole, etc.?
- Was the patient thrown from the car?
  - Was something in the car thrown against the patient?
- Was the patient ambulatory at the scene?
  - Did the patient need to be extricated from the vehicle?
  - How long did it take?
- Were there any other people in the car?
  - Were they injured?
  - What are their injuries?
- Was the pediatric patient in a car seat?
  - Where was the car seat located within the vehicle?
  - Was it struck by a deployed air bag?
  - Was the car seat strapped tightly with the seat belt?
- Were there law enforcement personnel at the scene?
  - If so, which agency?
- Does the patient wear:
  - contact lenses?
  - glasses?
  - hearing aid?
  - dentures?
  - Were they worn at the scene?
  - female patients: is a tampon in place?
- Where is the patient experiencing pain?
- Is the patient taking any medication, especially aspirin or other anticoagulants?
- Is there anyone the patient wishes to have notified?

---

5. Expose and examine:
   - ▲ undress the patient completely
   - ▲ provide for warmth and privacy of patient
   - ▲ assess neurologic status completely
D. Perform secondary survey and intervene as necessary.
   Once the quick primary survey is completed and life-threatening problems have been attended to, the ED team progresses to systematically performing a thorough assessment of the patient. Careful documentation is essential.
   1. Obtain complete set of vital signs.
   2. Assess general appearance.
      - ▲ body positioning
      - ▲ guarding

    ▲ body posture

    ▲ self-protection movements

3. Note any odors.

    ▲ gasoline

    ▲ urine

    ▲ feces

    ▲ alcohol

    ▲ chemical odors

    ▲ anything unusual

4. Perform head-to-toe assessment, checking for symmetry, deformity, discomfort, swelling, bleeding, and depression.

    ▲ head and face
  - bone deformities
  - soft tissue injuries

    ▲ neck
  - inspect
  - palpate

    ▲ clavicles and chest
  - bony deformities
  - soft tissue injury
  - expansion during ventilation
  - observe and auscultate breathing

    ▲ abdomen
  - distention
  - bruising
  - soft tissue injury
  - auscultate bowel sounds
  - palpate all four quadrants

    ▲ pelvis and genitalia
  - soft tissue injury
  - place hands on each side of the pelvis and gently squeeze inward to assess for tenderness, crepitus, instability
  - bleeding from the urethral meatus
  - rectal exam by the physician should always be performed *before* the placement of the Foley catheter

    ▲ extremities
  - soft tissue injury
  - sensory function
  - bony deformity
  - motor function
  - circulatory status
  - crepitus

    ▲ posterior assessment
  - maintain c-spine precautions
  - assist physician in log-rolling patient, utilizing ED team

▶ *Glasgow Coma Scale*

The Glasgow Coma Scale (GCS) is a method of quantifying a patient's state of consciousness (Table 2–30). It is an assessment tool used for patients with trauma, head injuries, headaches, etc. The accuracy of the GCS may be affected if the patient is hypoxic or hypotensive. It is important to use the GCS as a *part* of the patient's total assessment.

▶ *Trauma Score*

- ▲ This is an important field index that assists health care professionals in assessing the severity of the patient's injury (Table 2–31).
- ▲ The trauma score should be used on patients who do *not* have an obvious head injury.
- ▲ This tool assesses respiratory rate, respiratory effort, systolic blood pressure, capillary refill, and the GCS.
- ▲ A number is assigned to each finding and the total score is between 1 and 16.
  - ▲ A trauma score of 16 predicts a 99% survival rate, whereas a trauma score of 1 predicts a 0% survival rate (Table 2–32).
  - ▲ A score of less than 12 should be considered for immediate transfer to a level I trauma center.

▶ *Revised Trauma Score*

- ▲ The *revised trauma score* (RTS) is similar to the trauma score.
- ▲ It allows more weight to be given to the GCS and a more accurate assessment of the patient with an isolated head injury.
- ▲ A number is assigned to each finding (Tables 2–33 and 2–34).

TABLE 2–30 • Glasgow Coma Scale

	Infant (Preverbal)	Child/Adult
Eye opening	4 Spontaneously 3 To speech 2 To pain 1 No response	4 Spontaneously 3 To voice command or speech 2 To pain 1 No response
Best verbal response	5 Coos/babbles/cries appropriately 4 Irritable cry 3 Cries only to pain 2 Moans or grunts to pain 1 No response	5 Oriented 4 Confused 3 Inappropriate words 2 Incomprehensible words or vocal sounds 1 No response
Best motor response	6 Spontaneous 5 Localizes pain or withdraws to touch 4 Withdraws from pain 3 Abnormal flexion to pain (decorticate) 2 Abnormal extension to pain (decerebrate) 1 No response	6 Obeys commands 5 Localizes pain, purposeful movements 4 Withdraws from pain 3 Abnormal flexion to pain (decorticate) 2 Abnormal extension to pain (decerebrate) 1 No response
Total Score =		

TABLE 2–31 • Trauma Score

Physical Sign	Value	Points
Respiratory rate	10–24	4
	25–35	3
	>35	2
	<10	1
	0	0
Respiratory effort	Normal	1
	Shallow or retractive	0
Systolic blood pressure	>90	4
	70–89	3
	50–69	2
	<50	1
	0	0
Capillary refill	1–2 sec (normal)	2
	>3 sec (delayed)	1
	None	0
Glasgow Coma Scale	14–15	5
	11–13	4
	8–10	3
	5–7	2
	4	1
	3	0

TABLE 2–32 • Estimated Survival Rate Based on Trauma Score

Trauma Score	Survival (%)
16	99
14	96
12	87
10	60
8	26
6	8
4	2
2	0

TABLE 2–33 • Revised Trauma Score

Variable	Value	Points
Glasgow Coma Scale	13–15	4
	9–12	3
	6–8	2
	4–5	1
	3	0
Systolic blood pressure	>89	4
	70–89	3
	50–69	2
	1–49	1
	0	0
Respiratory rate	10–29	4
	>29	3
	6–9	2
	<6	1
	0	0

TABLE 2–34 • Estimated Survival Rate Based on Revised Trauma Score

Revised Trauna Score	Estimated Survival (%)
12	99
10	88
8	67
6	63
4	33
2	28

The total score will be between 1 and 12, with the estimated survival rate for each above.

> ## ◤ TRAUMA, MULTIPLE (PEDIATRIC)

▲ Pediatric trauma is a life-threatening situation that requires the ED staff to perform quickly and precisely.

▲ The smaller size of pediatric trauma victims predisposes them to a clinical status that can easily deteriorate.

▲ It is therefore essential that:
  • quick and accurate injury assessment occurs (consider using the Pediatric Injury Assessment Form)
  • treatment is quickly implemented
  • transfer to a Pediatric Trauma Center is implemented when appropriate
  • accurate documentation occurs

▲ Pediatric patients differ from adult patients in some ways, and it is important for ED nurses to understand those differences and prepare for them accordingly (Table 2–35).

❗ ALERT

- Children have greater oxygen demands and caloric requirements because of a higher metabolic rate.
- Children have highly reactive vascular systems that maintain systolic blood pressure in spite of blood loss. This sympathetic response to injury masks early signs of hypovolemic shock.
- Children can lose up to 25% of their circulating blood volume *before* a drop in their BP is seen.
- Children have immature and pliable skeletons that do not protect internal structures.
- Children are still growing, so any untreated injury may result in progressive or permanent deformity and disability.
- Airway compromise, hemorrhage, shock, chest injuries, and central nervous system injury are the leading causes of death in pediatric trauma victims.

 ### Assessment and Interventions

Upon notification of an incoming pediatric trauma victim, the ED team should prepare as in the *Multiple Trauma* guideline. However, special considerations exist for the pediatric patient, and the following modifications are essential in assessment and the interventions.

A. Perform primary survey and intervene immediately as necessary.

  1. Airway with cervical spine control:
     ▲ position head in a neutral, midline position
       • flexion or hyperextension of the neck may compress the airway in an infant due to the soft cartilage of the airway

  2. Breathing:
     ▲ assess for:
       • grunting
       • head bobbing

TABLE 2–35 • Pediatric Emergency Equipment

| Age and Weight | Airway/Breathing | | | | | Blood Pressure | Other | |
	Oxygen Mask	Bag–Valve Mask	Laryngoscope Blade	ET Tube	Suction Cath	BP Cuff	IV Catheter	Foley Catheter
Premie 1–1.5 kg	Premie Newborn	Infant	#1 straight	2.5 uncuffed	6–8 Fr	Premie Newborn	22, 24	5
0–6 months (newborn) 3.5–7.5 kg	Newborn	Infant	#1 straight	3.0 uncuffed	8 Fr	Newborn Infant	20, 22, 24	5
6–12 months 7.5–10 kg	Pediatric	Child	#1 straight	3.5 uncuffed	8–10 Fr	Infant Child	20, 22, 24	5, 8
1–3 years 10–15 kg	Pediatric	Child	#2 straight or curved	4.5 uncuffed	10 Fr	Child	18, 20, 22	10
4–7 years 17.5–23 kg	Pediatric	Child	#2 straight or curved	5.5 uncuffed	10 Fr	Child	18–20	10–12
>7 years >24 kg	Adult	Child Adult	#2 or #3 straight or curved	6.0 cuffed	10–14 Fr	Child Adult	16–20	10–12

- stridor
- prolonged expirations
- nasal flaring
- retractions

▲ count respiratory rate for full 60 seconds in infants <1 year old

▲ use blow-by O_2 when a conscious child rejects the oxygen mask

3. Circulation:

▲ insert two large-bore IVs (18–20 gauge/children, 20–22 gauge/infants)

▲ consider intraosseous infusion for children 6 years or under, if IV not in place within 90 seconds

▲ send blood samples to lab:
  - include type and screen, or crossmatch
  - perform bedside finger stick glucose test

▲ if child is in shock:
  - administer 20 ml/kg bolus of warmed NS or LR over 5 to 10 min
  - reassess patient
  - repeat fluid bolus if tissue perfusion remains inadequate
  - reassess patient
  - if shock continues after two fluid boluses, consider 10 mL/kg of warm packed RBCs (type-specific or O negative)
  - if blood is not available, consider albumin

> **! ALERT** A child in hypovolemic shock often requires at least 40–60 mL/kg of fluid in the first hour of resuscitation.

4. Disability:
   ▲ assess mental status

   A = **A**lert
   V = **V**erbal response
   P = **P**ain
   U = **U**nresponsiveness

   ▲ identify mechanism of injury (Tables 2–36 through 2–38)
   ▲ assign pediatric trauma score
B. Perform secondary survey and intervene as necessary.
   1. Expose and examine:
      ▲ briefly scan body
      ▲ undress patient
      ▲ initiate warming methods
         • warmed oxygen
         • warmed blankets
         • radiant warmer
   2. Vital signs:
      ▲ obtain respiratory rate, apical pulse, blood pressure
      ▲ obtain rectal temperature
   3. History (in addition to subjective data from Multiple Trauma guideline)
      ▲ immunization status
      ▲ for infants, determine birth history
   4. Head-to-toe assessment:
      ▲ head, face, and neck
         • infant anterior and posterior fontanelles detect fullness or bulging
      ▲ *Raccoon eyes:* periorbital ecchymosis that may indicate a head injury 12 to 24 hours old and a possible basilar skull fracture
      ▲ *Battle's sign:* ecchymosis over the mastoid area that may indicate an injury 12 to 24 hours old and possible basilar skull fracture
      ▲ chest, clavicles
      ▲ abdomen
         • may take 12 to 24 hours for intra-abdominal injuries to be obvious
      ▲ insert orogastric or nasogastric tube to decompress stomach
      ▲ posterior pelvis and genitalia
      ▲ extremities
      ▲ assessment (same procedure as with adults)

TABLE 2–36 • Mechanisms of Injury: Infant (Birth to 1 Year)

COMMON MECHANISMS OF INJURY
- Airway compromise
  - choking
  - strangulation
  - suffocation
  - foreign-body ingestion
- Child abuse
  - shaken-baby syndrome
- Falls
- Burns (scalds or flame)
- Drownings
- Poisonings
- Baby walkers
- Motor vehicle-related injuries
  - with or without the proper use/placement of car seats

Injury Pattern	Risk Factors	Associated Injuries
Head	Head large in proportion to body Poor head control due to weak neck muscles Pliable body structures and vessels predispose infant to diffuse head injury	Skull fractures: abuse, falls Subdural hematoma: abuse Retinal hemorrhages: abuse traumatic asphyxia Diffuse cerebral swelling: MVAs, abuse, falls High cervical fracture: MVAs

Chest	Tongue large in relation to oral cavity
	Narrow airway
	Obligate nose breather
	Short trachea
	Pliable rib cage
	Mobile mediastinal structures
	Absence of valves in superior and inferior vena cava
		Respiratory arrest:
		    airway compromise
		    foreign body ingestion
		    obstruction
		Pneumothorax: MVAs, falls, abuse
		Pulmonary/cardiac contusion: MVAs, falls

Abdomen	Pliable pelvic girdle does not protect internal organs
	Portion of bowel adheres to spine
	Organs easily crushed between bony structure and
	    injury object
		Laceration, fracture, rupture of solid organs
		    (liver, spleen, kidney): MVAs, abuse, falls
		Hematoma, perforation of hollow organs:
		    (esophagus, stomach, intestines): MVAs,
		    physical abuse

C. Document:
- ▲ initial assessment
- ▲ reassessments
- ▲ interventions
- ▲ serial vital signs
- ▲ input/output
- ▲ immunizations
- ▲ injury inventory (consider using Pediatric Injury Assessment form)

D. Transfer to pediatric trauma center:
- ▲ if facility is not a pediatric trauma center, consideration for higher level of care should be discussed and appropriate transfer arrangements implemented immediately.

TABLE 2–37 • Mechanisms of Injury: Toddler and Preschooler (1–6 Years)

COMMON MECHANISMS OF INJURY
- Motor vehicle-related injuries
  - occupant
  - pedestrian
  - bicycle
- Burns
  - scald and flame
- Drownings
- Ingestions
- Minor surface trauma
- Child abuse
- Firearms (preschoolers)
- Falls
- Sledding
- Choking
- Animals bites

Injury Pattern	Risk Factors	Associated Injuries
Head	Thin, pliable bony structures predispose diffuse cerebral injuries	Diffuse cerebral swelling: MVAs, falls Subdural hematoma: abuse, falls Skull fractures: MVAs, falls, abuse, sledding
Chest	Short trachea Compliant chest wall Mobile mediastinal structures Major vessels lack valves and predispose traumatic asphyxia	Pulmonary/cardiac contusions: MVAs, falls, sledding Pneumothorax: MVAs, falls, abuse Traumatic asphyxia: MVAs
Abdomen	Pliable pelvic girdle fails to protect internal organs Proportionately larger abdominal organs Ribs do not protect upper abdominal contents Organs are in close proximity to each other Portion of bowel adheres to spine	Laceration, fracture, hematoma to solid organs (liver, spleen, kidney): MVAs, falls, abuse Hematoma to hollow organs (esophagus, stomach, intestines): MVAs
Long bones	Epiphyseal plates do not ossify until puberty, may mask a fracture on x-ray (see Salter Harris Fractures Table 2–21) Periosteum is stronger and allows bone to bend, leading to greenstick fractures	Long-bone fractures: falls, MVAs, abuse, sports

▶ Pediatric Trauma Score

▲ The *pediatric trauma score* (PTS) is similar to the trauma score and the revised score.
  - Critical pediatric assessment areas are given special attention (Table 2–39).
▲ A number is assigned to each finding.
  - The total score ranges from no injury (12) to fatal injury (−6).
▲ A patient with a PTS range from 0 to 8 has increased chances of mortality.
  - A child should be cared for in a pediatric trauma center as soon as possible.

TABLE 2-38 • Mechanisms of Injury: School-Age and Adolescent (7–17 Years)

COMMON MECHANISMS OF INJURY
- Motor vehicle-related injuries
  - occupant
  - pedestrian
- Bicycle-related injuries
- Burns
  - flames
  - explosions
- Suicide
  - ingestion
  - gunshot wounds
  - hanging
- Minor trauma
  - superficial lacerations
- Drowning
- Falls
- Sports-related injuries
- Farm injuries
- Penetrating trauma
  - stabbing
  - gunshot wounds

Trauma	Associated Injuries
Motor vehicle accident	Head: cerebral swelling, epidural/subdural hematoma, skull fractures, c-spine injuries Chest: pulmonary/cardiac contusion, hemo/pneumothorax rib fractures Abdomen: liver—fracture, laceration 　　　　　spleen—hematoma, laceration, rupture 　　　　　kidney—hematoma, contusion, hematuria 　　　　　pancreas—contusion 　　　　　Misc: surface trauma, bony fractures
Bicycle	Head: closed or open injuries Chest: pulmonary/cardiac contusion, pneumothorax, rib fractures
Burns	Surface trauma, risk of multiple trauma exists
Drowning	Respiratory: acute respiratory distress syndrome (ARDS)
Falls	Head: cerebral swelling, epidural/subdural hematoma, skull fracture, c-spine injury Chest: pulmonary/cardiac contusion, hemo/pneumothorax Abdomen and misc: same as for motor vehicle accidents
Sports-related injuries	Head: c-spine injuries Chest: rib fractures, pulmonary/cardiac contusions Abdomen: same as MVA possibilities
Suicide	Head: c-spine injury from hanging Chest/abdomen: variety of injuries from penetrating trauma, falls, MVAs
Minor trauma	Surface trauma: lacerations, contusions
Penetrating trauma	Head/chest/abdomen: variety of injuries to internal organs
Assaults	Head/chest/abdomen: closed or open injuries, fractures, c-spine injury

TABLE 2–39 • Pediatric Trauma Score

Physical Indicator	Condition	Points
Airway	Normal	+2
	Maintainable with oral or nasal airway	+1
	Intubated or tracheostomy	−1
Weight	>20 kg (>40 lbs)	+2
	10–20 kg (22–44 1bs)	+1
	<10 kg (< 22 1bs)	−1
BP/Palpable pulse	>90 mmHg (+radial pulse)	+2
	50–90 mmHg (+femoral pulse)	+1
	<50 mmHg (no palpable pulse)	−1
Level of consciousness	Completely awake	+2
	Obtunded	+1
	Comatose	−1
Open wound	None	+2
	Minor	+1
	Major or penetrating	−1
Skeletal fractures	None	+2
	Closed fractures	+1
	Open/multiple fractures	−1

SKIN AND SURFACE TRAUMA (LACERATIONS, ABRASIONS, PUNCTURES, BITES, AMPUTATIONS)

Assessment

A. Obtain and record triage assessment that includes:
   1. Mechanism of injury
      ▲ mass and size of the wounding object
      ▲ velocity of the object and direction of impact
   2. Time of injury
   3. Blood loss
   4. Pain
      ▲ location
      ▲ quality
   5. Paresthesia, particularly distal to injury
   6. Immediate care of injured area
B. Assess wound for and document:
   1. Dimensions:
      ▲ size
      ▲ shape
      ▲ configuration
   2. Presence of:
      ▲ edema
      ▲ drainage
      ▲ deformity
      ▲ foreign body
      ▲ devitalized tissue
   3. Bleeding:
      ▲ oozing
      ▲ controlled
      ▲ pulsatile
   4. Range of motion distal to injury
C. Palpate (utilizing universal precautions) for:
   1. Pulses distal to injury
   2. Foreign body
   3. Underlying deformity
   4. Normal sensation distal to injury
   5. Lymphadenopathy proximal to injury
D. Remove *all* rings from *all* fingers of patients with hand, wrist, or forearm injuries.
E. Complete remainder of basic triage protocol and document accurately.

Interventions

1. Control bleeding.
2. Splint area if suspicion of bony injury exists, and order x-ray (if facility policy permits).
3. Obtain aerobic and anaerobic cultures from deep within the wound.
4. Remove hair around wound:
   ▲ clip with scissors
   ▲ do not shave hair from around wound (increases the risk of infection)
   ▲ *never* remove hair from the eyebrow
5. Cleanse wound.
   ▲ abrasions
     • must be cleansed thoroughly since skin layers may trap foreign particles, forming traumatic tattooing when the area heals
     • use a high-porosity sponge or soft surgical brush and a nondetergent cleansing solution for scrubbing
   ▲ lacerations
     • usually cleansed utilizing high-pressure irrigation with normal saline
   ▲ puncture wounds
     • cleansing technique varies depending on injury
   ▲ bite wounds
     • cleanse with high-pressure irrigation, with copious amounts of normal saline
   ▲ prepare for possible debridement of wound when necessary
     • assess for risk of rabies; may consider blood work if wound is obviously infected
   ▲ amputation
     • place amputated part in plastic bag, and place the bagged part in a container of ice
     • *do not* place amputated part directly on ice or in solution
     • provide wound care to stump
     • administer dT per ED protocol
6. Consider IV placement for antibiotic administration for:
   ▲ puncture wounds
   ▲ open fractures
   ▲ bite wounds
   ▲ amputations
7. See Box 2–10 for additional bite wound information.

■ Box 2–10: ADDITIONAL INJURY INFORMATION TO CONSIDER

1. Human bite wounds
   - High risk of infection
   - Occlusal bite wounds
     - laceration or crush injury to affected body part
     - human teeth marks on skin, ecchymosis, swelling
   - Clenched-fist injuries
     - occurs when a clenched fist strikes the mouth and teeth of another person
     - when hand relaxed from the fist position, the wound may appear to be sealed

2. Cat bites
   - 30%–50% of wounds become infected
   - Abscess formation
   - Risk of septic arthritis, osteomyelitis, sepsis
   - Infection develops <24 hours = gram-negative aerobe
   - Infection develops >24 hours = staph or strep

3. Cat-scratch disease
   - Small macule or vesicle develops into a papule
   - Low-grade fever, malaise, headache
   - Regional lymphadenopathy develops 3 weeks postinjury and resolves after 2–4 months

4. Dog bites
   - Risk of crush injuries, puncture wounds, and hand wounds
   - Fatal bites more common in small children, due to inability to protect themselves and due to exsanguinations from a major blood vessel
   - Assess for risk of rabies
   - Monitor closely for risk of infection

5. Black widow spider bites
   - Local reaction:
     - sharp, burning pain at the site within minutes of the bite
     - wound looks like two tiny puncture wounds from the fangs
     - tender skin that begins to blanch with surrounding erythema ("target lesion")
     - may *NOT* be able to see or palpate anything at the wound
   - Systemic reaction:
     - onset within 20–30 minutes
     - painful muscle cramps leading to clonic contractions
     - may have chest tightness, dyspnea, abdominal rigidity
     - agitation, tachycardia, shock

(*continued*)

■ Box 2–10: **ADDITIONAL INJURY INFORMATION TO CONSIDER** (Continued)

6. Brown recluse spider bite
   - Local reaction:
     - pain and induration leads to a blister formation with erythema
     - necrosis occurs in the area, and wound heals by secondary intention
   - Systemic reaction:
     - fever
     - nausea, vomiting, diarrhea
     - petechial or urticarial rash
     - acute renal failure
     - disseminated intravascular coagulopathy (DIC)
     - shock

7. Scorpion bite
   - Immediate onset of symptoms which progress to maximum severity within 5 hours
   - Erythema at area of wound
   - Sympathetic and parasympathetic stimulation
   - Seizures, respiratory failure

8. Jellyfish sting
   - Local pain and swelling
   - May progress to chest tightness, dyspnea
   - Tachycardia
   - Allergic reaction

9. Snake bites
   - Local:
     - puncture wounds with pain and swelling
     - involved extremity may become edematous, develop compartment syndrome
     - ecchymosis, petechiae, and hemorrhagic vesicles
   - Systemic:
     - weakness, diaphoresis, dizziness
     - severe bites can lead to cardiac dysfunction, renal failure, shock, respiratory distress

10. Tick bite
    - Attach to the skin, or burrow under it
    - May develop Rocky Mountain spotted fever or Lyme disease

PART III

Pearls of Triage Wisdom

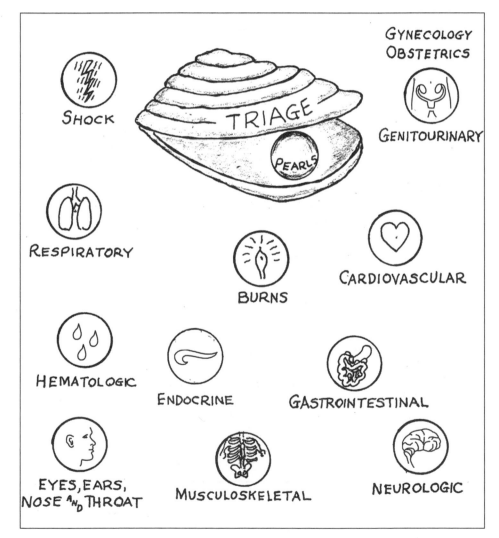

Notes

ASSESSMENT BY SYSTEMS

Table 3–1 illustrates assessment findings by various systems.

TABLE 3–1 • Assessment by Systems

System	Assessment Finding	Could Indicate

Respiratory	• Stridor, inability to talk
	• Mental status changes
	  • apprehension
	  • anxiety
	  • agitation
	  • confusion
	  • restlessness
	  • lethargy
	• Severe chest pain, guarded posture
		• Airway obstruction
		• Hypoxemia
		• Pulmonary embolus
		
		• Chest trauma

Cardiovascular	• Changes in
	  • skin color and temperature
	  • decreased or absent pulses
	  • pain
	• Hypotension
	• Oliguria
	• Decreased LOC
		• Vascular compromise
		
		• Decreased cardiac output

Neurologic	• Change in LOC • Bradycardia • Widened pulse pressure • Pupillary change • Paralysis or parenthesis	• First sign of neurologic deterioration • Increased ICP • Increased ICP • Brainstem injury • Cranial nerve damage • Brain injury • Spinal cord injury
Gastrointestinal	• Vomiting • Abdominal distention • Tachycardia • Hypotension • Diaphoresis • Pallor • Pain • Guarding • Rigidity	• Bowel obstruction • Ulcer • Internal bleeding • Internal bleeding • Hypovolemia • Peritoneal irritation
Musculoskeletal	• Deformity • Swelling • Decreased range of motion • Immobility • Bruising	• Fracture • Dislocation

TABLE 3–1 • **Assessment by Systems (Continued)**

System	Assessment Finding	Could Indicate
	• Poor capillary refill • Pallor • Cool skin • Absent or diminished pulses	• Vascular compromise
	• Paralysis • Numbness • Decreased sensation	• Nerve injury
Eyes, Ears, Nose, and Throat	• Limited extraocular movements • Decreased sensation • Facial asymmetry • Hearing or vision loss	• Neuromuscular damage
	• Local swelling • Redness • Drainage • Fever • Tenderness • Lesions	• Infection
	• Nasal or neck swelling • Stridor • Dyspnea • Tachypnea	• Respiratory compromise
Endocrine	• Dry mucous membranes • Decreased skin turgor • Hypotension • Tachycardia	• Dehydration • Hypovolemia • DKA • HHNC • Adrenal crisis
	• Alterations in LOC	• DKA • HHNC • Hypoglycemia
	• Tachypnea	• Hypermetabolism • thyrotoxic crisis
	• Bradypnea	• Hypometabolism • myxedema coma
	• Kussmaul respiration	• DKA
Hematologic	• Petechiae • Ecchymoses • Hematoma • Uncontrolled bleeding	• Coagulation disorder
	• Fever • Chills • Hypothermia • Signs of dehydration	• Sepsis
	• Progressively decreasing LOC • Shortness of breath • Tachypnea • Cyanosis	• Cerebral ischemia • Hypoxia due to decreased RBCs

TABLE 3–1 • Assessment by Systems (Continued)

System	Assessment Finding	Could Indicate
Gynecology and Obstetrics	• Tachycardia	• Internal bleeding
	• Cool, clammy, pale skin	• Shock
	• Restlessness	
	• Fetal bradycardia	• Fetal distress
	• Fetal tachycardia	
	• Hypertension	• Preeclampsia
	• Edema of the face or hands	
	• Proteinuria	
	• Apprehension	
	• Vertigo	
	• Generalized edema	• Eclampsia
	• Tonic–clonic muscle reflexes	
	• Convulsions	
	• Coma	
Genitourinary	• Ecchymoses in the flank area	• Retroperitoneal bleed
	• Severe colicky pain	• Renal calculi
	• flank	
	• abdominal	
	• groin	
Shock	• Altered mental status	• Decreased cerebral tissue perfusion
	• Tachycardia	• Decreased cardiac output
	• Tachypnea	• Poor tissue perfusion
		• Acidosis
	• Pale, cool, clammy skin	• Compensatory sympathetic response

LOC = level of consciousness; ICP = intracranial pressure; DKA = diabetic ketoacidosis; HHNC = hyperosmolar hyperglycemic nonketotic coma.

GERIATRIC PATIENTS

▲ The geriatric patient needs more time during triage since communication with older patients can be difficult.
  • The triage nurse must speak slowly and clearly.
▲ The triage nurse will need to determine how well the patient can hear, see, and speak.
▲ The triage nurse must continually assess not only the patient's physical and emotional condition, but also how well the patient understands the triage questions.

TABLE 3-2 • Structural and Functional Changes Resulting From Aging

Body System	Alteration
Tissues	Decreased number of active cells Reduced tissue elasticity
Cardiovascular	Decreased distensibility of blood vessels Increased systolic blood pressure Increased systemic resistance Decreased cardiac output Slow response to stress
Pulmonary	Decreased strength of respiratory muscles Limited chest expansion Decreased number of functioning alveoli Decreased elastic recoil, small-airway collapse Decreased resting oxygen tension Diminished protective mechanisms
Neurologic	Decreased number of functional neurons Decrease in nerve-conduction velocity Short-term memory loss Reduction in cerebral blood flow Decreased visual acuity and speed of dark adaptation Decreased pupillary response and accommodation Increased auditory tone threshold Diminished sensation and touch acuity
Gastrointestinal/Genitourinary	Decreased peristalsis Diminished acid secretion and thickened mucosa Decreased total nephron count Decreased glomerular filtration rate Diminished concentrating ability
Musculoskeletal/Integumentary	Narrowing of intervertebral disks Bone loss, increased risk for fractures Increased wear on joints Decreased number of muscle cells Loss of muscle strength Loss of skin thickness

▲ When necessary, the triage nurse may need to rely on family or friends who are present to provide pertinent information.

▲ Many elderly tend to complain less often than people in other age groups do.
  • The triage nurse should carefully evaluate for the possibility of elder abuse.

▲ The geriatric patient frequently takes several medications.
  • The triage nurse should carefully document *all* medications the patient is currently taking.
  • The nurse may photocopy a written list if the patient brings in one and attach it to the patient's chart.
  • Be sure to check for herbal supplements, over-the-counter medications, and illegal drug use.

▲ While assessing the patient, the triage nurse must remember that several factors influence the health of the geriatric patient.
  • Not all functional changes are related to disease.
  • Compensatory mechanisms decline with aging.
  • Injury/illness frequently occurs in "clusters."
  • There is increasing vulnerability to disease with aging.

▲ Aging also presents a challenge when considering drug absorption and distribution.
  • Slower absorption of oral and parental drugs
  • Slower absorption of drugs requiring acidic medium because of decreased acidity of gastrointestinal tract
  • Slower absorption of suppositories because of decreased blood supply to the rectum and lower body temperature
  • Slower drug distribution because of reduction of active and passive transport systems
  • Greater amount of pharmacologically active drug present because fewer plasma proteins are available for binding
  • Slower drug metabolism and longer duration of action resulting from decreased liver enzyme production, caused by decreased circulation to the liver
  • Increased concentration of drug resulting from decreased body mass and surface area and decreased renal function

▲ Table 3–2 lists the structural and functional changes resulting from aging.

▶ MENTAL HEALTH PATIENTS

▲ Triaging the psychiatric patient requires the nurse to be able to *sort through* the patient's medical and emotional needs (Table 3–3).

▲ The nurse needs to remember the following:

- Patients who present at the ED exhibiting aggressive and/or agitated behavior should be *considered violent until proven otherwise.*
- *Never turn your back* on a patient displaying aggressive or agitated behavior.
- Attempt to "talk them down" and seek additional help immediately.
- *Be simple, direct, clear, and concise* when speaking to the patient.
- *Remain calm* when dealing with an aggressive, agitated, hostile, or manic patient.
- Be careful *not to overlook* other physical injuries or illnesses in the psychiatric patient.

Patients who may be potentially violent include those with:

▲ history of substance abuse
▲ aggressive behavior
▲ verbal or physical threats of violence
▲ history of violent behavior
▲ history of childhood physical abuse
▲ suicidal or homicidal behavior
▲ presence of hallucinations or delusions
▲ presence of psychosis
▲ presence of organic, borderline, or antisocial personality disorder

TABLE 3–3 • **Mental Status Exam**

Area	*Assessment Considerations*
APPEARANCE	
	How does the patient look?
	Is he/she well groomed?
	How is he/she dressed?
ACTIVITY	
	Are there particular or unusual mannerisms?
	How is the patient's posture?
	What is the gait like?
	Is the patient agitated? Pacing?
AFFECT	
	Range of emotions *displayed* (happy, sad, unchanging, etc.)
	The patient may state he or she is happy, while appearing sad to others
	Does the patient look angry, sad, depressed, elated or nervous?
	Are expressions appropriate to actions or words?
	Are expressions labile and do they change quickly?
	Is it difficult to determine whether the patient is feeling anything?
	Is affect flat or blunted?

TABLE 3–3 • Mental Status Exam (Continued)

Area	Assessment Considerations
EYE CONTACT	Is the patient gazing with a fixed stare? Are the eyes darting about? Does the patient avoid eye contact with the triage nurse? Will the patient even open his eyes?
MOOD	The prevailing emotion felt The *feeling* the patient states he/she has ("I feel sad")
SPEECH	What is the rate of speech? Slow? Fast? What is the volume of speech? Is it clear? Is it slurred? Any strange speech patterns in how/what the patient is saying?
THOUGHT CONTENT	Topics of thinking and/or conversation Is the patient delusional? Is the patient hallucinating? Auditory? Visual? Olfactory? Tactile? What are the voices saying? Is the patient a threat to self or others?
THOUGHT PROCESS	Flow of conscious or mental activity as indicated by speech Are the patient's thoughts organized? Does the patient have a flight of ideas? Observe for rate, flow, associations, logical topics
ORIENTATION	Awareness of person, place, time, situation, relationships to other people

MEMORY	Does the patient have:
	    immediate recall?
	    recent memory?
	    remote memory?

INSIGHT	Is the patient aware of his or her own responsibilities and abilities? Is the patient able to analyze his or her area of concern objectively?
JUDGEMENT	Is the patient able to make appropriate decisions? Does the patient have good/fair/poor impulse control?

> ## OBSTETRIC PATIENTS

Physiologic Changes of Pregnancy

CARDIOVASCULAR

- ▲ Displacement of the heart by the enlarged uterus will produce ECG changes:
  - left-axis deviation of 15 degrees
  - flattened or inverted T waves in lead III
  - supraventricular ectopy may occur more easily
- ▲ Exaggerated splitting of the first heart sound, a loud, easily heard third sound
- ▲ Systolic murmurs are common and usually disappear after delivery.
- ▲ Maternal resting heart rate may increase as much as 15 bpm.
- ▲ Tachycardia refers to a heart rate >100 bpm.
- ▲ BP remains at prepregnant baseline or drops 5 to 15 mmHg.
- ▲ Maternal blood plasma volume increases 40% to 45% over prepregnant baseline.
- ▲ Maternal blood plasma volume at term is above 4000 mL.
- ▲ Increased blood plasma volume without increased blood cell mass results in a physiologic dilutional anemia of pregnancy (Hgb 11–13 gm/dL).
- ▲ Due to increased blood volume, clinical signs of shock will not appear until a woman has lost 35% of her total blood volume (~1400 mL).
  - Special attention must therefore be given during a trauma situation, since the early signs of shock may be blunted.
- ▲ Peripheral venous pressure rises in the lower extremities because of the weight of the pregnant uterus, while remaining unchanged in the upper extremities.
- ▲ Central venous pressure rises from 1 to 5 to 10 mmHg in the third trimester.
- ▲ In the supine position, the large uterus compresses the inferior vena cava, which results in decreased venous return from the lower half of the body to the heart.
  - This may cause arterial hypotension (supine hypotensive syndrome).
  - Venous return increases when the woman turns onto her left side.
- ▲ Increased cutaneous blood flow dissipates excess heat caused by the increased metabolism rate of pregnancy.

RESPIRATORY

- ▲ Increases occur in tidal volume (40%–45%) and minute volume (40%).
- ▲ Respiratory rate increases as oxygen consumption increases.
- ▲ Increased total volume lowers blood PCO_2 causing mild respiratory alkalosis, which is compensated by lowering of the bicarbonate concentration.
- ▲ The base of the thoracic cage is shortened and widened, while the diaphragm is elevated to allow for the enlarging uterus.
- ▲ Increased mobility of the rib attachments allows the thoracic cage to expand.

GASTROINTESTINAL

- ▲ Gums become hyperemic and softened, and may bleed easily.
- ▲ Heartburn easily occurs as a result of the stomach and intestines being displaced upward and laterally.

▲ Increased progesterone production by the placenta leads to decreased tone and motility of the GI tract that results in delayed gastric emptying and intestinal transit time.

▲ Hemorrhoids occur because of the increased venous pressure in the lower extremities and from constipation.

▲ Gallbladder may become distended as a result of decreased emptying time and the thickening of bile.

▲ Signs of peritoneal irritation are less reliable than in a nonpregnant woman.

▲ Abdominal rebound tenderness and rigidity are often diminished, delayed, or absent.

URINARY

▲ The ureters are compressed at the pelvic brim from the enlarging uterus, resulting in the dilatation and elongation of the ureters.

▲ Bladder is displaced superiorly and anteriorly, rendering it more susceptible to injury.

▲ Decreased serum creatinine (0.5 mg/dL) and BUN (10 mg/dL) occur later in pregnancy due to increased renal blood flow and glomerular filtration rates (GFR).

▲ Glucosuria may occur as a result of the increased GFR without increased tubular resorptive capacity for filtered glucose.

ENDOCRINE

▲ Slight enlargement of the pituitary gland

▲ Moderate enlargement of the thyroid gland
  • Basal metabolic rate increases up to 25% due to metabolic activity of the fetus.
  • Increased thyroxin and protein-bound iodine levels due to increased estrogen levels

▲ Increased adrenal secretions and aldosterone

▲ Alterations in maternal insulin production and usage occur due to fetal glucose needs for growth.

INTEGUMENTARY

▲ Increased levels of the melanocyte-stimulating hormone, beginning in the second month, produce changes in the woman's pigmentation.

▲ Striae gravidarum appear as reddish streaks on the abdomen, breasts, and thighs.

▲ Linea nigra is a dark brown line of pigmentation down the middle of the abdomen.

▲ Chloasma (mask of pregnancy) is seen as mottling of the cheeks and forehead.

▲ Angiomas (vascular spiders) may appear as small red elevations on the face, neck, upper chest, and arms.

▲ There is an increase in facial and body hair, a fine lanugo on the face and chest.

▲ Hair on the head may straighten, and an increase in hair loss may occur.

MUSCULOSKELETAL

▲ Hormonal changes increase the mobility of the sacroiliac, sacrococcygeal, and pelvic joints.

▲ The increased mobility of these joints may cause alteration in the woman's posture and lead to back pain and discomfort.

▶ **PEDIATRIC PATIENTS**

▲ *Listen* to the parents, *look* at the child.
▲ If a child is old enough to participate in meaningful verbal exchange with the triage nurse, then *look at* and *listen to* the child.
  • Don't hesitate to ask the child about his or her symptoms.
  • To develop a trusting relationship with the health care staff, the child must be made to feel important.
▲ Some children are good historians, some are not. Parents and guardians may provide the clarifying information when taking a pediatric history.
▲ Be patient when working with children.
  • Move swiftly when working with very sick or injured children, always maintaining a calm manner.
  • Avoid conveying panic to the child and the parent.
▲ Parents know their children better than anyone else!
  • If parents present at triage stating that "my child is not acting right," *listen* to their concerns.
  • This may be critical information that otherwise would be missed by the triage nurse.
  • Make NO ASSUMPTIONS that the parent(s) may be overreacting until organic issues have been ruled out.
▲ When caring for a pediatric patient, the triage nurse should also "care" for the parent or guardian of that child.
  • If the parent is anxious, the child will be too.
  • If the parent is angry, issues regarding the child's health may become clouded.
  • Offer support and education whenever possible.
  • Offer concern and care to the parent and address issues as they arise.
  • Ask a reflective question to the parent directly, such as: "You seem upset, is there something you would like to talk about?" The nurse may find out vital information by this sort of question.
▲ Allow children to make simple choices on their own, such as:
  • which arm to use for BP
  • what color Band-Aid to choose
  • whether to sit on parent's lap or in own chair
▲ Parents or guardian may underestimate the seriousness of illness or injury in the pediatric patient (e.g., sepsis).
  • Triage nurses must be keenly aware of the difference between parents' perceptions and sound nursing assessment of a patient presentation.
▲ Nonaccidental trauma or child abuse should be suspected with any child when there are conflicting histories.
▲ Obtain weights on all pediatric patients.
  • For uncooperative preschoolers or toddlers, weigh the parent and child together, then weigh the parent alone and subtract to find the child's weight.
▲ Count respiratory rate first, even before approaching or touching the small child.
  • This assures an accurate respiratory rate.
  • If the child is crying while counting the respiratory rate, document accordingly on the triage note (e.g., respiration 32/crying).
  • By documenting the child's behavior, subsequent respiratory rates can be better interpreted.
▲ Respiratory rates in children less than 1 year old must be counted for a full minute.

■ Box 3–1: CIAMPPEDDS

C = Chief complaint?
   Why did you bring the child to the ED?
I = Immunizations?
   Are the immunizations up to date?
A = Allergies?
   Is this child allergic to any medications?
M = Medications?
   Does the child take any medications on a regular basis?
P = Past medical history?
   Is there a history of past illnesses, injuries, or hospitalizations?
P = Parental impression?
   What is different about your child now that prompted you to bring him or her to the ED?
E = Events surrounding the child?
   Has anyone else at home or school been sick?
D = Diet?
   Is the child eating (nursing) well?
D = Diapers?
   How many wet diapers in the past 8 hours? Is this a usual amount?
S = Symptoms?
   What symptoms have you seen with this current illness or injury?

- Infants have a naturally irregular pattern of breathing and must therefore be evaluated for a full minute to accommodate for this irregularity.
▲ Do all painful or invasive procedures last if possible. When painful procedures are done before simple ones, the child may distrust or fear all subsequent treatments and interactions.
▲ Consider using the Emergency Nurses Association mnemonic for pediatric assessment, **CIAMPPEDDS**, Box 3–1.

Differences in the ABCs

AIRWAY

▲ Children have large tongues and their airway can be easily obstructed.
   - Proper positioning may be all that is necessary to open the airway.
▲ Airways have much smaller diameters and can be easily obstructed by small amounts of mucus or swelling.
▲ The cartilage of the larynx is softer than in adults, and the infant airway can be compressed if the neck is flexed or hyperextended.

BREATHING

▲ Sternum and ribs are cartilaginous and intercostal muscles are poorly developed, causing the infant's chest wall to move inward instead of outward during inspiration (retractions) when lung compliance is decreased.
▲ Infants are obligate nose breathers for the first 6 months of life.
   - Anything causing nasal obstruction can produce respiratory distress.

TABLE 3–4 • Pediatric Vital Signs: Normal Ranges

Age Group	Respiratory Rate	Heart Rate	Systolic Blood Pressure	Weight	
				Kilograms	Pounds
Newborn	30–50	120–160	50–70	2–3	4.5–7
Infant (1–12 months)	20–30	80–140	70–100	4–10	9–22
Toddler (1–3 years)	20–30	80–130	80–110	10–14	22–31
Preschooler (3–5 years)	20–30	80–120	80–110	14–18	31–40
School-age (6–12 years)	18–25	70–110	85–120	20–42	41–92
Adolescent (13+ years)	12–20	55–110	100–120	>50	>110

Remember:
- The patient's normal range should always be taken into consideration.
- Heart rate, BP, and respiratory rate are expected to increase during times of fever or stress.
- Respiratory rate of infants should be counted for a full 60 seconds.
- In a clinically decompensating child, the blood pressure will be the **last** to change. Just because your pediatric patient's BP is normal, don't assume that your patient is "stable."
- Bradycardia in children is an ominous sign—usually a result of hypoxia. Act quickly since this child is extremely critical.

CIRCULATION

▲ Pediatric patients have a circulating blood volume that is larger per unit of body weight.
  - Blood loss considered minor in an adult may lead to shock in a child.
  - A decrease in fluid intake or increase in fluid loss can quickly lead to dehydration.
▲ Tachycardia is a pediatric patient's most efficient method of increasing cardiac output and is the first sign of shock.
  - Cardiac output decreases if heart rate is greater than 180 to 200 bpm.

Normal Vital Signs

Table 3–4 lists normal pediatric vital sign ranges.

Abnormal Vital Signs

Table 3–5 lists several abnormal vital signs.

TEMPERATURE: HYPERTHERMIA

▲ Infants under 12 weeks of age with a fever of greater than 100.4°F rectally should be evaluated immediately.
▲ They are less capable of localizing infections than older children.
▲ These infants may harbor a serious bacterial infection while appearing benign.
▲ Bacterial infections must always be ruled out, including:
  - bacteremia
  - otitis media
  - meningitis

TABLE 3–5 • Abnormal Pediatric Vital Signs

Age	Respiratory Rate	Heart Rate	Systolic Blood Pressure	Urine Output (Normal = 1–2 mL/kg/hr)
Newborn	<30 >50	<120 >160	<50 >70	<2–6 mL/hour
Infant (1–12 months)	<20 >40	<80 >150	<70 >100	<4–20 mL/hour
Toddler (1–3 years)	<20 >30	<80 >140	<75 >110	<10–28 mL/hour
Preschooler (3–5 years)	<20 >30	<80 >120	<80 >110	<14–36 mL/hour
School-age (6–12 years)	<18 >25	<70 >120	<85 >120	<20–44 mL/hour
Adolescent (13+ years)	<12 >20	<55 >110	<90 >120	<30–50 mL/hour

- urinary tract infection
- pneumonia
▲ The most common causes of elevated temperatures in children are:
  - viral illness
  - gastroenteritis
  - upper respiratory infection

TEMPERATURE: HYPOTHERMIA

▲ Infants have unstable temperature-regulating mechanisms, a high body surface area-to-weight ratio, and quickly become hypothermic as a result of exposure.
▲ Hypothermia can lead to:
  - metabolic acidosis
  - bradycardia
  - decreased respiratory rate
  - cardiopulmonary arrest
▲ Sepsis and shock can lead to hypothermia.
▲ *Every attempt should be made to keep all infants warm.*

HEART RATE: TACHYCARDIA

▲ Common causes are:
  - fever
  - stress
  - anxiety
  - early shock

- ingestion of a chemical substance
- supraventricular tachycardiac (SVT)

HEART RATE: BRADYCARDIA

▲ *Bradycardia in children is always an emergency condition.*
  - Bradycardia may be signaling impending arrest.
  - Supplemental oxygen should always be provided.
  - Maintain ABCs.
▲ Other causes of bradycardia could be:
  - hypotension
  - acidosis
  - drug ingestion

! **ALERT** Bradycardia equals **hypoxia** until proven otherwise.

RESPIRATORY: TACHYPNEA

▲ Common causes are:
  - fever
  - stress
  - poisoning
  - dehydration
  - respiratory distress
  - CHF (in children with congenital heart disease)
  - diabetes
  - ketoacidosis

RESPIRATORY RATE: BRADYPNEA OR APNEA

▲ Common causes are:
  - shock
  - acidosis
  - hypothermia
  - poisoning
  - respiratory failure

BLOOD PRESSURE: HYPERTENSION

▲ Common causes are:
  - increased intracranial pressure
  - cardiovascular disease
  - drug ingestion
  - renal disease
  - endocrine disorders

BLOOD PRESSURE: HYPOTENSION

▲ Common causes are:
  • shock (a late sign)
  • drug ingestion

TABLE 3–6 • Suggested Immunization Schedule: 2002								
Immunization	*Birth*	*2 Months*	*4 Months*	*6 Months*	*12–15 Months*	*4–6 Years*	*11–12 Years*	*Adult*
Hepatitis B	X	X			X			
Diphtheria, pertussis, tetanus (DPT)		X	X	X	X	X		X (dT)
H. influenza type b (HIB)		X	X	X	X			
Inactivated polio		X	X		X	X		
Measles, mumps, rubella (MMR)					X	X		
Varicella					X			
Pneumococcal conjugate (PVC)		X	X	X	X			
Influenza				X (yearly)				

PART IV

Enhanced Triage: Beyond the Basics

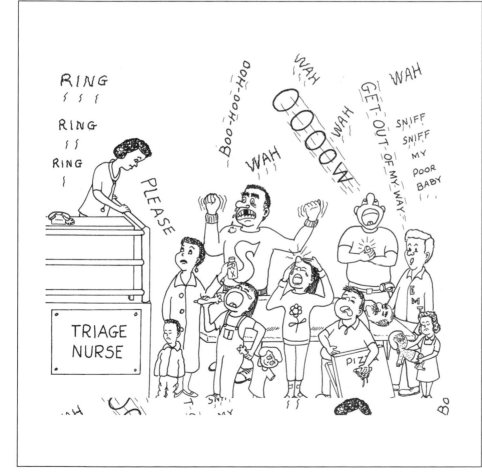

Notes

Triage is a specialized skill that is developed on an individual level, at an individual pace of growth. While a nurse may be in the triage role with only a few years of experience, the knowledge of a "seasoned" triage nurse is equivalent to a thousand pages of text. This chapter will share some of those lessons learned by nurses throughout years of triage experience—with the goal that newer nurses won't have to learn *everything* the hard way.

► CROSS-CULTURAL EMPATHY

The triage nurse encounters a large variety of patient presentations, some life-threatening and others relatively insignificant. All require professional expertise and care. When the triage nurse greets and assesses the persons requesting care, ethnic, religious, cultural, or social similarities are found between the patient and the nurse. Some qualities of each patient are similar to those of the triage nurse and some differ. It is essential for the triage nurse to care for the patient and family without seeing differences as right or wrong, but simply different.

❗ ALERT   The celebration of difference is the next step beyond mere tolerance or acceptance.

Diversity Among Patients

Culture is a broad term used to describe:

▲ intellectual development of enlightenment, determination, and heritage that has occurred with the evolution of familial generations
▲ style, beliefs, traditions, and knowledge passed from one generation to another
▲ the sum total of creativity, inspiration, and philosophy of a group of people within a similar belief system

Diversity is a term used to describe:

▲ recognition that people are different from one another
▲ different ways people engage in cultural practices that are different in origin or purpose
▲ understanding that we are free to celebrate differences without judgmental bias of right and wrong

As a health care professional, the nurse must understand that any differences that are not fully examined will influence the outcome of the health care delivered. For health-promoting behaviors to be successfully developed, the relationship between the patient and nurse must be based on the acceptance that each person has the freedom to choose whether or not to behave in an established manner (McGregor & Barnet, 2002).

The health care professional is in a position to:

▲ act as a culturally informed educator
▲ be sensitive to the fact that a patient's belief system may influence his or her acceptance and compliance with the prescribed or recommended health care
▲ act as a role model for others who are unfamiliar with such patient diversity

The seasoned health care professional portrays confidence, friendliness, patience, and a gentle demeanor to assist the patient in coping with fear of the unknown and the uncertainties surrounding the ED visit. By offering a warm and welcoming feeling to *all* patients, the triage nurse increases patient satisfaction and compliance with prescribed health care services.

On the following pages are brief descriptions of diverse backgrounds, belief systems, and social circumstances patients may live by on a day-to-day basis. It is important, however, to remember that these are generalizations and may (or may not!) apply to your patient—**don't assume your culturally diverse patient practices identically to what you may read in any book.**

AFRICAN AMERICAN

▲ African Americans are one of the largest of the many racial and ethnic groups in the United States.
▲ They had been one of the most focused-on minorities until the 1990s, when affirmative action rulings began to emphasize all groups, minorities, and the disabled.
▲ Many families have a strong, extended family kinship.
▲ Grandmothers often play a strong role in the raising of grandchildren, especially when there is a single parent.
▲ Many African Americans are actively involved in church life, including numerous types of religions and belief systems.

AGNOSTIC

▲ This group neither believes in nor denies the existence of a God, believing that the evidence to prove or disprove God's existence is incomplete.

AMISH

▲ This is an ethno-religious group whose members live mostly in Ohio, Indiana, and Pennsylvania, as well as parts of the West and Midwest.
▲ They are a conservative offshoot of the Mennonites.
▲ Most Amish are farmers, use no electricity, have no telephones, and use manually powered farm equipment.
▲ Their central belief rejects worldliness and materialism; their style of dress is uniform and plain to avoid any pretext of vanity.
▲ Good mental and physical health are believed to be gifts from God, and hard work, a pure lifestyle, and a well-balanced diet contribute to good health.
▲ Worship is typically done at home, not in churches.
▲ They are stoic people and often refuse health care.
▲ Historically, they believe that immunizations are unnecessary, and death is regarded as the entrance to a better life.
▲ Most feel that life-support technology is inappropriate.

ATHEIST

▲ Atheists believe that faith in a *God* who directs human destiny, who hears and responds to prayer, and who loves and cares for his creation is unwarranted by either test of scientific evidence or rational analysis of human experience.
▲ The importance of each person's own credibility is stressed, as is reliance on individual knowledge to explain life events.

▲ Atheists believe in neutral yet very powerful natural powers.

▲ Atheists may be devoutly spiritual.

▲ Patients may request the presence of others, significant to them, during crisis to provide human comfort and a sense of peace.

BAHA'I FAITH

▲ This is an independent religion with 5.4 million followers worldwide.

▲ Central teachings include oneness with God, religion, and humankind.

▲ Baha'is believe in harmony between religion and science.

▲ When ill or injured, they will seek modern health care from providers they trust, and pray.

BUDDHIST

▲ Buddha (c. 563 BC–c. 483 BC), who was known as the "Enlightened One," taught his followers how to achieve nirvana (inner peace) through morality, meditation, and wisdom.
  • He taught that community peace could be attained through example, such as quality role models.

▲ Buddhists believe that bad situations are often transitory and use their belief system to help overcome fear, anxiety, and apprehension.

▲ Patients may believe that crisis is a result of a wrong committed in the present or a past life (karma).
  • Many believe that if they are good, good will be done to them or a positive outcome will be their reward.
  • Kindness from providers is a comfort.

▲ Buddhism descends from Hinduism; many practices and concepts are shared by both communities.

CHRISTIAN SCIENCE

▲ Christian Science was founded in 1862 by an invalid woman who was miraculously healed after hearing an inspirational speaker profess that disease was merely an error of the mind.

▲ Believers seek to reinstate the original Christian message of salvation from all evil, sickness, disease, and sin.

▲ Health is restored by the principal belief of divine harmony, and adherents choose spiritual healing rather than medical care.
  • They may be aided with prayers for healing by Christian Science practitioners, identified individuals within the church who devote themselves to assisting believers with the process of spiritual healing through study of the Bible.

CUBAN AMERICAN

▲ Immigration to the United States began in 1959, when Fidel Castro took over the government of Cuba, and has not ceased since then.
  • Early immigrants were well-educated professionals. That began to change in the 1980s with the Mariel boat lift.
  • Cuban refugees then began to include dangerous and hard-core criminals, political prisoners, and those from the poor and less educated areas of Cuba.

▲ Cuban Americans are spread throughout American society in both city environments and suburban areas.
  • Their inability to return to Cuba has made their hold on their cultural past weaker than in other Hispanic communities.

▲ Cuban Americans have become active participants in American culture and tend to be active in politics, continuing education, entertainment, and sports.

FILIPINO AMERICAN

▲ Filipino Americans combine medical therapies with folk remedies.
  • Disease is associated with total life situations and with both natural and supernatural causes.
  • Spices are believed to have special healing powers.

GYPSY

▲ Diseases are divided into nongypsy (*gaje*) diseases, which are treatable by Western practitioners, and gypsy diseases (*drabarni*), which must be treated by their own practitioners.
▲ Disease is sometimes thought to be caused by the "evil eye."
▲ Some foods thought to be lucky and necessary for good health are:
  • pepper
  • salt
  • vinegar
  • garlic
  • onions
▲ Family presence is vital to reduce fear and anxiety.
▲ The "family" may comprise more than one "wife."
  • The term "wife" refers to a relationship of duty or obligation.
  • There may be several "wives," yet this is different than polygamy.
  • For legal purposes, verify the family and patient's definition of "wife" before obtaining authorization for patient care.

HAITIAN

▲ Haitians are immigrants from the mountainous island of Haiti, located in the Caribbean.
  • Although the island is shared with the Dominican Republican, they have little in common.
▲ Most Haitians speak a Creole patois, a mixture of French, Spanish, and English.
▲ The predominant cultural heritage retains its African roots.
  • Santeria, the primary religion, is a combination of Catholicism and African voodoo.
  • Haitians may use rituals of dance, music, magic, and cults of the dead for healing.
▲ Amulets, charms, or herbs may be used or worn in prayer for preventing or curing evil or illness.
  • Health care professionals should understand that removing these charms may create an emotional crisis for the patient and family; they should only be removed after careful consideration and discussion with the patient.
▲ Haiti is the poorest country in the Western Hemisphere.
  • Malnutrition among the rural poor is high, and malaria, tuberculosis, and hepatitis are common.
  • Health care is difficult to obtain, with one physician for every 30,000 rural inhabitants.

HINDU

▲ This common Indian religion evolved over several thousand years and intertwined history with the social system of India.
▲ Hinduism has no founder, no prophets, no set creed to follow, and no particular institutional structure.
▲ Hindu beliefs may be theistic or nontheistic and include:
  • reincarnation
  • karma
  • natural moral law
  • duty to follow within a divinely ordered society

▲ Domestic rituals occur for:
- birth
- puberty
- marriage
- death

▲ Hindus number more than 400 million worldwide.

HISPANIC

▲ This term refers to persons with a native language of Spanish, a specific national origin, and a shared cultural background.

▲ Included in this group are:
- Mexican Americans
- Dominican Republic immigrants
- Central and South Americans
- Puerto Ricans
- Cubans

HOMELESS

▲ Few social problems have increased as suddenly or been dramatized as effectively as the plight of the homeless during the 1980s and 1990s.

▲ At one time, the homeless person was invisible and ignored by mainstream Americans.

▲ Currently, the homeless can be seen anywhere and may include:
- "bag ladies" wandering the streets with their worldly possessions in a bag
- men sleeping at the side of buildings
- runaway or throwaway children scrounging for food and shelter
- drug addicts
- working poor individuals and families who cannot afford housing

▲ The National Institute of Mental Health has estimated that one third of the homeless are former mental patients who have been discharged under deinstitutionalization programs.

▲ Many homeless are addicted to drugs or alcohol, and common practice now includes the exchange of sex for drugs.

▲ Health issues among the homeless are staggering, and include:
- untreated chronic illnesses
- rampant communicable diseases
- difficulty in finding affordable health care

▲ Public health agencies find it difficult to keep up with this very transient population.

ISLAM

▲ Followers of Islam are known as Muslims or Moslems, and their beliefs embrace every aspect of life.

▲ This religion originated in Arabia during the 7th century through the prophet Muhammad.
- Common belief is that all individuals, societies, and governments should be submissive and obedient to the will of God (Allah).

▲ It is the world's third greatest monotheistic religion, with more than 700 million followers.

▲ Islam emphasizes success, believing that it meets all of humankind's religious and spiritual needs.

▲ Daily prayer habits include praying five times a day while facing East.

▲ Dietary rules exclude the consumption of pork.
  • Fasting is a part of certain holidays.
▲ Some patients may choose to pray before medical interventions.
▲ Because of extreme modesty, Muslims may request to have a health care provider of the same gender as the patient.

JAINISM

▲ Originated from the Indus River Valley civilization of 3000 BC.
▲ There is not one all powerful God. Instead, there were 24 great teachers in the 6th century BC who preached to the people.
▲ They believe in reincarnation until peace and full knowledge is attained, at which time their soul will rest in the heavens forever (Nirvana).
▲ Principles include:
  • vegetarianism
  • nonviolence in thought, deed, and action

JEHOVAH'S WITNESS

▲ This religion was organized in the United States in 1884.
  • Their literal translation of the Bible differs from that of Protestants and Catholic churches.
▲ Witnesses believe Armageddon (the final struggle between the forces of righteousness and evil) and the second coming of Christ are near.
  • Jehovah's Witnesses believe they will be the only ones to endure the Armageddon.
▲ Worldly involvement is avoided; Jehovah's Witnesses do not participate in nationalistic ceremonies and do not celebrate holidays by gift giving.
▲ No distinction is made between clergy and laity, and patients may request that members of their religious group be present to comfort and talk with them.
▲ Most are *absolutely opposed* to blood transfusions.

JUDAISM

▲ There are varying degrees of religious orthodoxy and personal preferences regarding religious practices.
  • Observance of the Sabbath (from sundown Friday through sundown Saturday) may be strict.
▲ Two key figures provide guidance, leadership, and education:
  • rabbi: the primary spiritual leader
  • hazan (cantor): the artistic and spiritual role model who provides worshipers with the awe-inspiring chanting of the liturgy.
▲ Modern medicine is readily accepted.
  • Comfort for illness is often found through eating (e.g., chicken soup).
  • Some may follow strict traditional dietary laws. (Kosher meats tend to have a high sodium content.)
▲ Most are opposed to autopsy.
▲ Burial should take place within 24 hours of death whenever possible.

MENNONITE

▲ Mennonites evolved from Dutch and Swiss Anabaptists, who emphasized adherence to the word of the Scripture, strict church discipline, and the separation of church and state.

▲ The Anabaptists were the forerunners to both the modern-day Mennonites and the Baptist Church.

▲ Mennonites possess a deep concern for the individual's dignity and self-determination.

• Their belief system is similar to the Amish.

• Mennonites may accept modern medicine, immunization, and life-support techniques.

MEXICAN AMERICAN

▲ 86% of Mexican Americans reside in the southwestern United States, in search of a desirable lifestyle.

▲ This group of people is a product of historical development that began more than 4 centuries ago; they are the second oldest component of American history.

▲ In the past 50 years, they have emerged as a distinct and visible group.

• Most live in urban areas and share common problems with the rest of this country's urban poor.

▲ There has been an organizational movement since 1985; there are now more than 2,100 Mexican-American elected officials in this country.

▲ Strong importance is placed on family and extended family.

• Role obligations are seen as mandatory.

▲ For those who have migrated to the United States without their extended family, the loss of that social, emotional, and economic support may be a major stressor during time of illness.

MIEN

▲ This ethnic group transcends several religious customs and religious groups.

▲ They are often Christians if living in the United States, but may have a mix of Taoism and other Eastern religions for their practice.

▲ *Sip mien mien* are missionaries who perform ceremonies.

▲ Cupping is a common practice.

MIGRANT WORKER

▲ These are persons who move around in seasonal patterns looking for work.

▲ Migrant labor arose largely as a response to industrialization.

▲ As cities, offering factory jobs, expanded, people left farms for higher-paying work.

• The crops, however, still needed to be harvested.

• The lure of higher wages to people who saw no chance of improvement in their homelands pulled them toward more prosperous surroundings.

MORMON (LATTER-DAY SAINTS)

▲ Mormonism was founded in 1830 in the state of New York.

▲ Sacred books include the *Book of Mormon* and the *Doctrine and Covenants*.

▲ A common belief is that God was once a child, and that someday believers may also become gods.

▲ Bishops are considered spiritual leaders of the smallest unit of believers.

• They provide spiritual comfort during times of crisis, as well as advocate and arrange for the physical and social needs of the patient and family.

• The "laying on" of hands is used as part of their divine healing.

▲ Most do not use alcohol, illegal drugs, tobacco, or caffeine.

NATIVE AMERICAN

▲ This is a term used for the indigenous people of North, Central, and South America, covering a wide range of languages, habits, ethnic origins, and religions.

▲ Migration for survival (hunting, cultivating) and competition with the expanding white population led to great dislocation, reaction, and interaction within the various groups and with Christianity.

▲ Most Native American religious systems recognize a cultural hero, employ themes from Christianity, and stress inherited traditional spirituality.

PENTECOSTAL

▲ This is a modern-day Christian renewal movement that began in Kansas in 1901.
  • This group practices a literal interpretation of the Bible, with informal worship services and enthusiastic participation by all.

▲ There are more than 22 million followers worldwide, and since the 1960s, it has appeared within the established Protestant, Catholic, and Greek Orthodox churches.

▲ Pentecostals believe in divine healing through prayer.
  • Anointing with oil may be practiced with laying on of hands.
  • Some believe illness is divine punishment, but most consider illness an intrusion of Satan.

▲ Deliverance from sin and sickness is provided for by praying for divine intervention in health matters, and members seek to reach God through prayer for themselves and others when ill.

▲ Most Pentecostals abstain from pork, alcohol, and tobacco.

PROTESTANT

▲ This is a generic term used to describe the belief in the Christian faith that evolved from the Reformation as a protest against Roman Catholicism in 1515.
  • The individual believer, not only the clergy, is seen as credible.

▲ There are many denominations, including Adventist, Baptist, Episcopal, Lutheran, Methodist, and Presbyterian.

PUERTO RICAN

▲ As a result of the Spanish-American War, Puerto Ricans are U.S. citizens by birth.
  • Many have settled in cities in the Northeast after leaving the island of Puerto Rico because of poor economic conditions and high unemployment rates.
  • There is a two-way migration pattern between the island and the mainland, and many find employment as seasonal workers along the East Coast and in the Midwest.

QUAKER

▲ This Christian sect was founded in 1667.

▲ This group believes that God is in every person and can therefore be approached directly.

▲ Religion is seen as a personal, inward experience.

▲ Simplicity is emphasized in all things; followers are active promoters of tolerance, justice, peace, and often are conscientious objectors during wartime.
  • An example of Quaker belief commitment occurred in the early 18th century, when they played a significant part in the abolition of slavery.

ROMAN CATHOLIC

▲ Believers of Christian doctrine, *the people of God*.
  • Church doctrines have remained largely untouched since its beginning, and followers accept the traditions as authoritative.
▲ The Vatican (an independent state in Rome), under the direction of the Pope, implements policy and controls this vast and complex organization.
▲ Principal doctrines include God as trinity, redemption, creation, the *place* of the Holy Spirit, and the *person* and the *work* of Jesus Christ.
▲ It is important to understand that Catholics may believe that the souls of infants who die unbaptized will not be able to enter heaven.
  • Any lay person may baptize an infant with a sprinkle of water, saying "I baptize you in the name of the Father, Son, and Holy Ghost."
▲ Some critically ill patients may request to have a priest called to administer the Sacrament of the Sick.
  • Having access to a prayer book or rosary beads may bring comfort.

SEXUAL ORIENTATION

▲ Characteristics of human sexuality involve biologic, psychological, and sociologic behaviors.
  • Sexual orientation is complex and has been studied and included in every civilization throughout history.
▲ An individual's affiliation with a particular religious, social, ethnic, or cultural group may be influenced by the group's attitudes that may allow, encourage, or condemn a person's right to choose a sexual identity other than adult heterosexuality.
▲ A person's right to choose is monitored and lobbied for by numerous civil rights groups in the United States.
  • Equal opportunity in employment, housing, business, and health care is sought and obtained.
  • The courts become involved when issues of discrimination based on sexual orientation arise.

SIKHISM

▲ A progressive religion, founded more than 500 years ago
▲ Has a following of more than 20 million people worldwide and currently ranked as the 5th largest religion
▲ Beliefs include:
  • devotion and remembrance of God at all times
  • truthful living
  • equality of mankind
  • denouncement of superstitions and blind rituals
  • some followers who never cut their body hair
  • strict avoidance of tobacco, alcohol, or drugs
    – however, some militant groups of Sikhs are known for their heavy use of hashish
  • wearing of a turban as a symbol of royalty and dignity

SOUTHEAST ASIAN (CHINESE, CAMBODIANS, INDOCHINESE)

▲ People who belong to this group may believe that illness is a result of weak nerves, imbalance of *yin* and *yang*, an obstruction of *chi* (life energy), disharmony with nature, a curse, or as a punishment for immorality.

▲ Coining, cupping, burning, pinching, and moxibustion may be practiced.

▲ Herbal remedies are commonly used.

▲ Trust and security rarely extend beyond the family.

▲ Most are sensitive to social class distinctions, and modesty may require caregivers and translators be of the same gender as the patient.

▲ They may speak at least one of the following: Vietnamese, Cambodian, Laotian, or Hmong (a Laotian tribal language).

▲ *Amulets* are simple black strings with several large knots and are worn around the wrist, waist, or neck.
  • They represent prayers for preventing or curing evil or illness.
  • Health care professionals should understand that removing an amulet may create an emotional crisis for the patient and family.
  • It should be removed only after careful consideration and discussion with the patient.

VIETNAMESE

▲ Immediate and extended families are extremely valuable.
  • Mothers generally care for children for the first 2 years of life, after which paternal grandmothers assume much of the responsibility.

▲ Religions practiced include a combination of:
  • Buddhism
  • Confucianism
  • Taoism
  • Roman Catholicism

▲ Health concepts are heavily influenced by their religious beliefs, including:
  • illness results from a bad deed in this or a previous life
  • a balance between *yin* and *yang* forces maintains immunity and prevents disease
  • possible refusal to have blood drawn for lab tests since it is believed that losing blood depletes the body's strength and provides a route for the soul to leave the body
  • possible refusal of blood transfusions since they give the opportunity for another person's spirit to enter the patient's body

YUGOSLAVIAN (FORMER)

▲ Bosnia, Croatia, Herzegovina, Macedonia, Serbia, Slovenia
  • As a result of the civil war and political conflict in the former Yugoslavia, terrible tolls have been exacted on adults and children.
  • Most health care resources have been focused on survival.
  • Routine care of chronic illnesses, health maintenance, and care for the young has been nonexistent.

▲ More than 17,000 children have died since the beginning of the war.

▲ Persons surviving the war are experiencing an increase in:
  • devastating mental health illness
  • mortality for common health issues
  • complications of routine congenital defects, injuries, and chronic illnesses
  • infant mortality
  • birth defects

Common Cultural Healing Practices

▲ A common belief is based on the premise that the body is composed of:
- air
- fire
- water
- earth

▲ These components of the body have the characteristics of:
- hot
- wet
- dry

▲ To prevent sickness and maintain good health, traditional practices occur which often include:
- herbal remedies
- tonics
- avoidance of excesses in life
- massage
- procedures based on hot/cold physiology

▲ The ED staff must assess carefully, as some of these practices will leave marks on a patient's body that may be mistaken for abuse.

▲ Table 4–1 describes specific cultural practices that are commonly used to treat ailments.

TABLE 4–1 • Common Cultural Practices

Practice	Treatment for	Process	Appearance
Burning	Pain Cough Diarrhea Failure to thrive	A dried weed is dipped in hot lard, ignited, and applied to the skin.	Asymmetric, superficial painful burns on the forehead, neck, front or back of the body
Coining/Rubbing	Fever Pain "Colds" Vomiting Headache Muscle cramps	The edge of a smooth metallic coin or spoon is dipped in menthol oil and rubbed vigorously downward over the symptomatic area. Often used over the chest, back, shoulders, and neck areas.	Superficial ecchymotic areas that typically occur in a striped pattern May appear as parallel linear marks on or near the spine, ribs, trachea, or upper arms May look like the person was "whipped" This is the most commonly practiced remedy method.
Cupping	Fever Headache Cold Cough Dizziness Pain	The inside of a glass is coated with rubbing alcohol. The glass is heated and placed on the skin where a vacuum forms. The cup is left in place for up to 30 minutes on the trunk, shoulder, abdomen, or forehead.	Symmetric flat, circular ecchymotic areas Appear on chest, abdomen, back, or forehead May be painful to touch The number of areas produced can indicate the severity of the patient's symptoms and/or the length of the current illness.
Hair pulling	Headache	The hair is pulled in an attempt to stop a headache.	Patches of hair may be missing if the hair was pulled with too much force.

TABLE 4–1 • Common Cultural Practices (Continued)

Practice	Treatment for	Process	Appearance
Moxibustion	Abdominal pain Diarrhea Ulcers Hernia	The moxa herb is rolled into a pea-sized ball and placed on the skin. The ball is then lit and allowed to burn to the point of pain.	Often resemble cigarette burns May be in a pyramid shape Appear on the abdomen, chest, or back
Pinching	Headache Cold/flu Pain Fever Heat exhaustion Fainting Stomachache Vomiting Diarrhea	Skin is lubricated with mentholated ointment and massaged before pinching occurs.	Small welts or ecchymotic areas in a regular pattern May be seen in a pattern of 2–3 vertical rows on the neck, face, forehead, trachea, chest, upper arms, spine, or back
Stick burns	Fever Abdominal pain	A stick (similar to an incense stick) is lit and placed on the palms of the hands, the soles of the feet, or the genital area. In some cultures, a hollow bamboo stick stuffed with cotton is lit and then extinguished, then placed on the above areas of the body.	Circular, cigarette-type burns to the skin
Suctioning	Headache	The cut end of a bull or goat horn is placed on the patient's forehead and/or temple area. A small hole is bored into the pointed end of the horn, and the practitioner sucks the air out of the horn. The horn sticks to the site and the hole is then plugged with wax. The horn is left in place for about 15 minutes.	The blood is drawn to the surface of the skin and a round mark is left after the horn is removed. An ecchymotic bruise in the shape of the end of the horn remains on the body for several days.
Sweeping (with an egg)	Fever Headache Restlessness Crying Vomiting	Egg may be rolled on the body to pick up evil or demons and is then used to transport them away. Egg may also be used in a ceremony near the patient's bed.	Often no visible signs of this treatment
Sweeping (using orange, lemon, or palm leaves)	Anorexia Fatigue Insomnia Hallucinations Weakness	A healer (often a grandmother) uses branches or leaves to sweep over the patient's body while reciting prayers.	An herbal tea may be administered after this procedure. May not leave any physical marks on the patient May account for a delay in seeking modern health care

Natural Alternative Herbal Medicines

Years ago, our grandmothers would give us tea made of some leaf from her garden in an attempt to cure whatever ailed us. In today's world, more interest and belief is surfacing about the use of natural herbal supplements as an alternative method of caring for our health needs.

Whether you are a believer or not, our patients may be. It is important that as health care providers, we open up conversation to include the patient's use of herbal supplements.

Some supplements may adversely react with the prescribed medication from the physicians, so it is important that we better understand what our patients may be using (Table 4–2).

TABLE 4–2 • Natural Alternative Herbal Medicines

Herb or Substance	Uses	Side Effects	Interactions and Clinical Concerns
Acidophilus	Restores normal oral, GI, and vaginal flora in those affected by antibiotics, *Candida*, and bacterial infections	None reported	No significant toxicity has been reported.
Cascara (*Buckthorn, chittem bark, sacred bark*)	Laxative	Diarrhea Electrolyte imbalance with long-term use	Contraindicated in Crohn's disease Chronic use may cause melanin pigmentation of the mucous membranes of the colon.
Dandelion (*lion's tooth*)	Diuresis Appetite stimulant Dyspeptic complaints Liver/gallbladder disorders Regulation of blood glucose	Hypoglycemia Contact dermatitis	Acute toxicity risk is low May potentially be toxic because of high content of potassium, magnesium, and other minerals Do not use for empyema or obstruction of the bile ducts.
Echinacea (*black susans, comb flower, hedgehog, snakeroot*)	Topical wound healing Internal stimulation of the body's immune system	None reported	Long-term use not recommended Contraindicated in progressive disorders such as MS, collagenosis, HIV, AIDS, tuberculosis
Elderberry (*sweet elder, sambucus, common elder*)	Used in flavorings Diuretic Laxative	Nausea/vomiting Weakness Dizziness Numbness Stupor	Do NOT apply to the face of an infant. Overdose may lead to cyanide-induced toxicity, especially if stems and leaves are consumed.
Ephedra (*Ma-huang, yellow horse, popotillo, sea grape*)	Relieves "cold" symptoms Improves respiratory function Headache Anti-inflammatory agent	Palpitations Cardiac arrhythmia Depression (children) Nervousness Headache Insomnia Dizziness	CNS stimulant Do not use with MAOI antidepressants— combination may cause hypertensive crisis. Do not use with cardiac glycosides, anesthetics, guanethidine, vasoconstrictor sympathomimetics, oxytocin, beta blockers, or in patients with glaucoma. Uterine contractions, bronchodilation, diuresis

TABLE 4–2 • Natural Alternative Herbal Medicines (Continued)

Herb or Substance	Uses	Side Effects	Interactions and Clinical Concerns
		Anxiety Vomiting Hypertension	Hypoglycemia/hyperglycemia Use with caution in patients with hypertension or diabetes.
Eucalyptus	Rheumatic complaints	NA	May weaken the potential of other medication if taken together Do not use in patients with inflammatory bowel disease or bile duct problems.
Flaxseed (*Flax, lint bells, linum, linseed*)	Topical demulcent and emollient Laxative Cough and "colds" Urinary tract infections	None	Possibility that in large amounts there may be a cyanogenic concern, but this seems to be more with veterinary than with human medicine
Garlic (*Allium, stinking rose, rustic treacle*)	Lowers blood sugar, lipids, and cholesterol Antiseptic Antibacterial	Nontoxic but can cause oral and GI irritation Use with care in diabetics and those patients on anticoagulants	Inhibits platelet aggregation and increases fibrinolytic properties Use with caution in patients on anticoagulants. May increase serum insulin levels and decrease serum glucose levels
Ginkgo (*Kew tree, yinhsing, maidenhair tree*)	Raynaud's disease, anxiety Cerebral insufficiency, stress Tinnitus, dementia, memory Circulatory disorders, asthma Concentration	Severe side effects are rare Headache Dizziness Heart palpitations GI reactions Rash (resembles poision ivy)	Inhibits platelet-activating factor—bleeding episodes may occur Avoid use during pregnancy and lactation. Avoid eating the female fruit raw—causes contact dermatitis and ulcers.
Ginseng	Fatigue and irritability Lowers cholesterol Stress	Breast tenderness Nervousness Decreased concentration Lowers blood sugar	Contraindicated in patients on anticoagulants, taking stimulants (even caffeine!), antipsychotic drugs, or while being treated with hormones Use with caution in diabetics, those with cardiac problems, hypotension, hypertension, receiving steroids, pregnant woman, lactation. May potentiate the action of MAOIs
Glucosamine (*Chitosamine*)	Antiarthritic	Well tolerated No known side effects	No documented toxic effects Possibility of broncho-pulmonary complications
Golden seal (*Eye balm, Indian dye, orange root*)	Eyewash Antispasmodic Dysmenorrhea Minor sciatica Rheumatoid and muscular pain Traveler's diarrhea	Lowers blood sugar Nausea, vomiting Diarrhea Hypertension Seizures Respiratory distress	Contraindicated in diabetics or anyone taking anticoagulants Can cause cardiac excitability May cause local ulcers—do NOT use as a douche Causes uterine contractions—avoid use during pregnancy

TABLE 4–2 • Natural Alternative Herbal Medicines (Continued)

Herb or Substance	Uses	Side Effects	Interactions and Clinical Concerns
Hawthorne (*Haw maybush, whitehorn*)	Regulates blood pressure and heart rhythm Atherosclerosis and angina pectoris Antispasmodic Sedative	Nausea Fatigue Sweating Rash on the hands Hypotension Sedation	Increases the ejection fraction of the ventricles Increases the activity of cardiotonics such as digitalis Reduces uterine tone and motility—avoid using during pregnancy and lactation
Horse chestnut (*Chestnut*)	Edema, inflammation, and venous insufficiency Skin cleanser	Seeds of this plant are toxic. FDA classifies this as an "**unsafe**" herb. Twitching Dilated pupils Vomiting/diarrhea Depression Paralysis Stupor	Carcinogenic when used in skin cleansers Poisoning easily occurs when consumed as tea—death occurs rapidly. Nasal cancer occurs if horse chestnut pollen or dust is inhaled over a period of time.
Kava (*Awa kew, tonga*)	Local anesthetic Sedative Sleep aid	Dry, flaking, discolored skin Scaly rash Red eyes Puffy face Muscle weakness CNS depression	Contraindicated in pregnancy and lactation Avoid other CNS stimulants or depressants. High doses result in anorexia, low protein levels, increased HDL, hematuria, decrease platelet counts, hypertension.
Licorice	Settles an upset stomach Expectorant	Muscle weakness Lowers potassium level Hypertension Edema Glucose intolerance Uterine contractions	Side effects worsen for patients with underlying renal, hepatic, gallbladder, or cardiovascular disease or those patients receiving cardiac glycoside therapy or steroid therapy.
Melatonin	Regulates sleep Protects against cancer	Headache Depression	No significant toxicity has been reported.
Peppermint	Seasoning Flavoring Irritable bowel syndrome Abdominal pain	Contact dermatitis Flushing Headache Heartburn Bradycardia	Use with caution if patient has hiatal hernia (peppermint relaxes the esophageal sphincter, thus potentiating esophageal reflux). Contraindicated in pregnancy because of its emmenagogue effect, and in gallstones because of its choleretic activity
Saw palmetto (*Sabal, cabbage palm*)	Management of prostate enlargement Alopecia Asthma Indigestion	Headache Diarrhea	Do not use if pregnant or lactating.

TABLE 4–2 • Natural Alternative Herbal Medicines (Continued)

Herb or Substance	Uses	Side Effects	Interactions and Clinical Concerns
Soy (*Soya, soybean*)	Source of fiber, protein, and minerals Anticancer effects Alleviates menopausal symptoms Prevents osteoporosis Combats cardiovascular and GI problems	Soy dust may induce asthmatic attack.	No significant toxicity has been reported.
St. John's Wort (*Goatweed, Rosin rose*)	Depression	Rash Photosensitivity Tachycardia	Contraindicated with prescription antidepressants Take with food to prevent GI irritation. Contraindicated in pregnancy because of its emmenagogue and abortifacient effects—also causes uterine stimulation

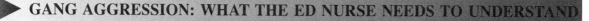

► GANG AGGRESSION: WHAT THE ED NURSE NEEDS TO UNDERSTAND

Rules to Remember

RULE #1

- ▲ The reason a gang member comes to the ED is for the same reason other patients come to the ED—they are sick or injured.
  - They do NOT come to the ED for drugs or violence. They can get *those* on the street.
- ▲ Gang members do not come to the ED to steal equipment.
  - They do not understand what the machines are for or what they are worth.
    - Without that knowledge, those items are useless when trying to sell stolen goods on the street.

> **! ALERT**   The primary reason a gang member comes to the ED . . . is PAIN !

RULE #2

- ▲ If the ED staff ever forgets **Rule #1**, then the ED staff is "behind the eight ball" for violence.

RULE #3

- ▲ If you forget that you are the best health care provider this gang member has ever seen or ever will see, you have then begun the process toward a possible altercation or other threat of violence.

There are many different types of people who come through the ED who pose a threat of violence to the ED staff. Believe it or not, gang members are less likely to create a scene in your ED than perhaps the common drug abuser or psychotic patient (as long as you follow the three rules listed above!). If the nurse is an expert in customer service, then there is little chance of the staff member irritating a potentially threatening person to the point of aggression towards the ED staff.

Gang members, however, may be less predictable than others prone to hostile acts. The more the staff understands about the "gang culture," the less chance of the ED staff provoking a violent incident with a gang member.

> **! ALERT**   To keep the ED safe while a gang member is present, always remember *what they are in the ED for (injury/illness)*, and *what they want (relief)*.

History

The first known organized gang dates back to 1826, which formed in the back of a little grocery store in New York City. They protected their territory from citizens and law enforcement officials and grew to be an expert group of pickpockets and thieves.

Over the years, gangs continued to develop. Groups of people with similar backgrounds, interests, and needs found safety and security in gang membership. Those reasons continue into today's societies. The reasons for joining a street gang today include:

- ▲ a sense of identity
  - which opposes societal norms
- ▲ a source of recognition
  - a sense of "being better" than others
  - because they lack character, integrity, and discipline, society has rejected them
  - therefore, they develop their own standards, cliques, method of acceptance
- ▲ a way of belonging
  - this gives them power, which they couldn't have through normal integrity and discipline in society
- ▲ established boundaries and discipline
  - this is another way of making their mark, letting others know that they "are tough"
- ▲ a basis of brotherhood or family
  - in their own perverted ways, this is their support system of people who care
  - it is the closest they will ever come to feeling the love of a family
- ▲ a source of money
  - being a gang member is all about drugs, sex, and alcohol
  - they have failed in modern society, so they "make their living" off the street

Gang Culture

While the most important thing for an ED member to remember about a gang member has already been stated, it may also help to be sensitive to the gang's mentality and gang culture. To do that, you must first understand the "Three Rs":

1. They want and expect to keep their **REPUTATION** ("rep").
   - ▲ This is a critical concern for gang members ("gangbangers").
   - ▲ A "rep" extends to each individual, as well as to the whole gang.
   - ▲ Status is achieved by one's "rep" and the history of past deeds and actions.
   - ▲ The more a gang member has accomplished, the higher his status within the gang.
   - ▲ When they are injured, they must show others that they can withstand the pain and anguish of being shot, stabbed, cut, etc.
   - ▲ The gang member must always be seen by others as being "brave."
2. They expect and at times will demand **RESPECT**.
   - ▲ Respect is sought for the individual gang member, as well as the gang as a whole, family members, and territory.
   - ▲ Respect is a VERY important part of being a gang member, and they work hard to keep their respect intact.
   - ▲ Gangs may intentionally show disrespect ("dis") for another gang through hand signals, graffiti, or by staring at them ("mad dog").
   - ▲ Health care providers should remember to NEVER call a gang member a wimp, or even imply it with facial expression.
   - ▲ Treat their positions with great care, including their jewelry, ornaments, and headwraps—mishandling them will be seen as a sign of disrespect towards the gang member.

If the health care provider *looks* at a gang member with an expression of disrespect, that gang member may become hostile and seek revenge for the lack of respect from the health care provider.

3. They will give you **RETALIATION AND REVENGE** if you fail to give them respect or threaten their reputation.
   ▲ It must be understood that in gang culture, *NO* challenge goes unanswered.
   ▲ Many drive-by shootings and other acts of violence follow an event of perceived disrespect.
   ▲ Commonly, a gang member perceives an incident of disrespect, leaves the area, and returns at a later time (hours, days, weeks) with his entire gang to retaliate and keep his reputation intact (Grossman, McNair, 2003).

A gang that seeks revenge upon a member of the ED for perceived poor treatment of their gang member may return hours, days, or weeks later to take revenge upon the entire ED staff.

Gang Identity

GROUPS

Many gangs exist in today's American societies. There are two major-league gangs, known as the Folks and the People.

   ▲ These leagues, like baseball and football leagues, are divided into individual teams (gangs) such as the famous Bloods (Red) and Crips (blue).
   ▲ Each gang has its own color.
   ▲ There are gangs of white men, female gangs, and gangs formed by immigrants from every country in the world.

The ED staff does NOT have to know the specifics of each gang, but must understand that gangs are different from each other and that they harbor an intense rivalry with other gangs.

COLORS, SYMBOLS, AND SPORTS TEAMS
   ▲ Gangs use colors, symbols, jewelry, tattoos, graffiti, and sports team clothing to identify themselves.
   ▲ If the nurse has a particular question about a patient's tattoo (or other symbol), he or she should simply ask the patient about it.
   ▲ **Remember to NEVER pass judgment on the patient's use of symbolism.**

ALERT   Use caution when working with gang members—ask their preference if there is a color choice (e.g., casting material)—and under NO circumstances ever place a person wearing a red bandanna near a person wearing a blue bandanna!!

GANG LANGUAGE

▲ There are different hand signals that the members may use to communicate with each other, as well as a vocabulary of their own. See Table 4–3 for examples of gang slang.

Staying Safe While on Duty

So, how do you stay safe while working in an ED?

▲ Focus is everything.
- Focus only on **WHY** they are in your ED and **WHAT** they want.
- Avoid judging them or thinking about their way of life.

TABLE 4–3 • Gang Language

Slang Term	Meaning
AB	Aryan Brotherhood
Academy	Prison or jail
Ace Kool	Best friend, backup
Always and forever	Blood for life
Be down	Loyalty, defend during adversity
Be real	Prepare for war
BIH	Burn in hell
Bitch	A sucker; someone that shows disrepect
BLA	Black Liberation Army (terrorist group)
Bomb	Marijuana laced with heroin
Body Shop	Clinton Correctional Facility (NY)
Boned out, book, break	To chicken out, to run away
BOSS	Brothers of the Steady Struggle
Bro	Brother, friend
Candy Land	Green Haven Correctional Facility (NY)
Cap	To shoot at
Click up	To get along with
Cola	Parole officer
Come with power	Bring your gang; a gang fight
Contract	A homicide
Da projects	Sing Sing Prison
Dead presidents	Money
Death Row	New York City
Deuce and a half	25-caliber semiautomatic pistol
Dime	10-year prison sentence, $10 bag of drugs
Dis	Disrespect
Dog	Gun
Doing a jack	Robbing someone
Double deuce	22-caliber gun
Drinking 40s	Drinking 40-ounce bottles of malt liquor

TABLE 4–3 • Gang Language (Continued)

Slang Term	Meaning
Expect rain (or thunder)	Expect trouble
Fila	Knife
Four Five	45-caliber semiautomatic gun
Free air	Released from prison
G-ride	Stolen vehicle
Game	Criminal activity
Ham sandwich	Derogatory term for Muslims
Juice	Power
Kite	Illegal written prison correspondence; a letter
Locs	Dark sunglasses
Looking to machine	Seeking sex
Make a move	Commit a crime
Mad dog	Dirty look
Mecca	Harlem, NY
Mushroom	An innocent bystander in a drive-by shooting
Pop goes the weasel	To kill someone
PoPo	Police
Pork chopper	Police helicopter
Red zone	Prepare for war
Seeing-eye nigga	I've got your back covered
Snow cone	Ice pick used as a weapon
Vida loca	Crazy life
Wet 'em up	To make someone bleed by stabbing or shooting them
Zip gun	Homemade pistol

▲ Show respect.
- Be confident in your care and always show respect.
- As professionals, we should be doing this naturally—it is especially important when working with gang members.
- Make each patient believe you are the best health care provider he or she has ever had.

▲ Knowledge is important.
- Knowledge is important to everyone.
- Gang members have their own language, hand signals, symbols, colors, etc. These things constitute "their knowledge."
- Health care professionals have their own knowledge.
- Talk health care language in a nonpatronizing manner for them to understand what is happening while they are under your care.

▲ Recognize the dignity of each individual.
- Each person has his or her own standard of dignity.
- Do not judge others by your personal standards.

! ALERT   Remember—gang members come to the ED because they are injured or sick and want to get better. Deliver your care by understanding the importance of *RESPECT*, *REPUTATION*, and *REVENGE*.

> ## BODY ART

Decorating the body is one of the earliest known forms of artistic expression. Body decorations were (and still are) used to:

- ▲ indicate a religious devotion
- ▲ protect from evil and disease
- ▲ camouflage against enemies
- ▲ identify with a particular tribe, culture, gang, or society
- ▲ enhance beauty of men and women
- ▲ attract members of the opposite sex
- ▲ celebrate passage from childhood to adulthood

Body Piercing

Piercing can be traced through history to Rome in 200 AD. The genitals of slaves and athlete were commonly pierced—slaves so that they would not reproduce, and athletes so that they would not waste athletic energy having sexual contact.

Prince Albert (1819–1861) was well known for having a piercing through his urethra, called a "dressing ring" by 19th century tailors (it was used to secure his genitalia to either the left or right pant leg).

For those who do not have a body piercing, it may come as an enigma as to "why" people would do this to themselves. Only the person who has a piercing can know for sure. The first time pierced genitalia is seen by a health care professional may be a shock.

Infections are a risk with any body piercing and are more common with piercings around the mouth, the nose, and the navel. Whenever possible, leave the jewelry in the piercing since this will allow a channel of drainage. Common organisms include:

- ▲ *Staphylococcus aureus*
- ▲ Group A beta hemolytic *Streptococcus*
  - • leads to endocarditis and glomerulonephritis
- ▲ pseudomonal infections
- ▲ hepatitis B
- ▲ hepatitis C
- ▲ HIV
- ▲ syphilis

When a patient presents to the ED for emergent care, the ED staff must be prepared for the special care these patients may need. Included are:

- ▲ if a piece of jewelry must be removed to provide care:
  - • ask the patient's permission
  - • learn about that particular piece of jewelry, as they all work a little differently from one another (see the section below on Body Piercing Jewelry)
  - • do **NOT** use a ring cutter to remove piercing jewelry since this will create rough edges that will damage the soft tissue when the jewelry is removed
  - • the hole can be preserved by inserting suture material through most pierced holes and tying a loose-looped knot

▲ c-spine:
  • stabilization may be difficult if there is piercing jewelry on the cheeks, chin, throat, or neck
▲ MAST trousers:
  • remove pierced genitalia and navel jewelry before application
▲ Sager splint:
  • remove pierced genitalia jewelry before application
▲ Foley catheter
  • insertion may be complicated if piercing goes through or near the urethra
▲ defibrillation/cardioversion
  • avoid placing paddles directly on the jewelry in the nipples or chest (no need to remove jewelry before procedure)
  • for chest implants that are superficial, long thin metal—there may be complications with this procedure

Body Piercing Jewelry

There are certain pieces of jewelry that must be used when piercing particular areas of the body (Figure 4–1).

CAPTIVE BEAD RING

▲ The ring does not have a bead attached to either end.
▲ The bead is held in place by the tension from both sides of the ring.
▲ The bead is inserted and removed by slightly opening the ring and relieving the tension on the bead.

BEAD RINGS

▲ A bead is permanently attached to one end of the ring.
▲ The ring is opened/closed by inserting/removing the free end of the ring in/out of the bead coupling.

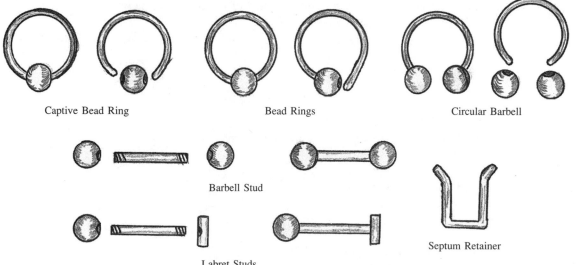

Captive Bead Ring   Bead Rings   Circular Barbell

Barbell Stud

Labret Studs   Septum Retainer

Figure 4–1. Jewelry used for body piercing.

CIRCULAR BARBELLS

▲ These rings have balls attached to both ends.
▲ The balls are threaded and removable by unscrewing the ball.

BARBELL STUDS

▲ These are straight bars with balls attached to each end.
▲ One or both of the balls are threaded and removed by unscrewing the ball.

LABRET STUDS

▲ These straight bars have a ball screwed on at one end and a flat disc screwed to the other end.

SEPTUM RETAINER

▲ This "U"-shaped piece of jewelry is inserted into a nasal septum piercing to preserve the hole when the person chooses not to wear noticeable jewelry. (It is undetectable when flipped up into nostrils.)

IMPLANTS

▲ Placement may occur almost anywhere on the body.
  • Head, neck, chest, extremities, genitalia
▲ Objects of Teflon, stainless steel, or other items are placed under the skin through small incisions.

Locations of Body Piercings

There are many places on the body that, if they have a "fold of skin," may be pierced (Figure 4–2).

AMPALLANG

▲ A barbell stud is placed horizontally through the head of the penis, normally above the urethra.
▲ Enhances the sexual pleasure of the woman

CHEEK

▲ May be located anywhere on the cheek

CLITORIS

▲ Can only be pierced if $\frac{1}{4}$" wide
▲ May be pierced horizontally or vertically through the center of the clitoris

CLITORIS HOOD

▲ May be pierced horizontally or vertically
▲ Found to be sexually stimulating

EARLOBE

▲ The most common piercing performed
▲ Seen as most socially acceptable
▲ Single or multiple piercings are evenly spaced and centered on the earlobe.

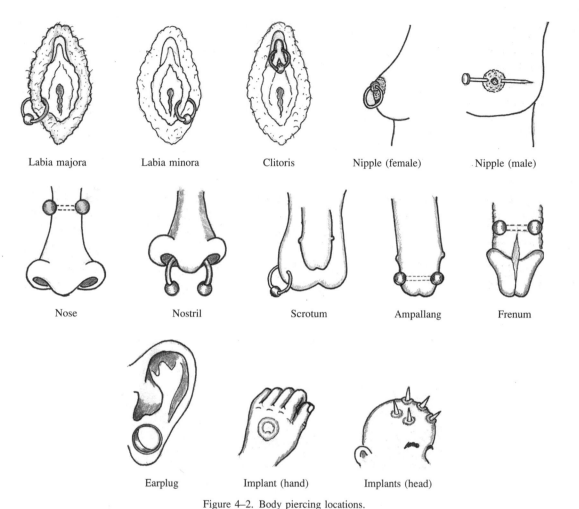

Figure 4–2. Body piercing locations.

EAR CARTILAGE

- ▲ Popular piercing location
- ▲ May be placed anywhere along the ear through the cartilage

EARPLUG

- ▲ The earlobe is pierced, and a small object is placed in the lobe.
- ▲ The object stretches the earlobe and is then replaced with a larger object.
- ▲ In time, an ear plug is placed into the lobe.

EYEBROW

- ▲ Popular location for piercing
- ▲ Piercing may occur anywhere along the length of the eyebrow.
- ▲ Normal piercing is vertical or angled slightly to the side.

FORESKIN

▲ Located near the leading edge of the foreskin when the penis is flaccid
▲ May have multiple piercings of this area
▲ Heightens sexual stimulation

FRENUM

▲ Located on the center underside of the penis where the glans meets the shaft
▲ May have multiple piercings of this area evenly spaced along the underside of the penis

HAND WEB

▲ Located in the flesh between the thumb and index finger
▲ Rarely done since it inhibits free use of hand

LABIA MAJORA

▲ Placement is along the leading edge of the outer labia lips.
▲ Often multiple pierced sites are placed in this area.
▲ Enhances erotic feelings

LABIA MINORA

▲ Placement occurs along the leading edge of the inner labia lips.
▲ Often multiple piercings are done in this area.
▲ Enhances erotic feelings

LIP

▲ Popular in many tribes around the world
▲ May be placed anywhere along the lip line, on the top or bottom lip

NASAL SEPTUM

▲ Piercing occurs through the thin tissue between the inner cartilage and the outside edge of the septum.
▲ The ring should hang freely if piercing is performed correctly.

NAVEL

▲ Only pronounced inward navels are suitable for piercing.
▲ Placement is 3/8" above the upper edge of the navel.
▲ The ring should hang vertically and appear to disappear into the navel opening.

NIPPLES (FEMALE)

▲ Considered attractive and sensual, while allowing the nipple to become larger and more pronounced
▲ Located at the base of the nipple where it meets the plane of the breast
▲ Should NOT go through the areolae

NIPPLES (MALE)

▲ Considered attractive and sensual, while allowing the nipple to become larger and more pronounced
▲ Usually piercings are placed into the areolae, unless the nipple is large.

NOSTRIL

- ▲ Common in many cultures
- ▲ Placement occurs in the crease formed where the lower edge of the nostril curves upward and forward around the base of the nose.

SCROTUM

- ▲ May pierce any area on the scrotum
- ▲ Piercings must be superficial without penetrating the scrotal sac.

TONGUE

- ▲ Very popular in today's culture
- ▲ Piercing occurs one inch from the tip of the tongue along the center line, in between the two large veins of the tongue.
- ▲ See Table 4–4 for common complications.

TRAGUS

- ▲ Placement should be in the natural fold where the tragus attaches to the side of the face.

Tattoos

- ▲ The history of tattoos date back to the 5th century BC.
- ▲ Common in today's culture
- ▲ There are two ways to obtain a tattoo:
  - professional artist with an established studio, with electric tattoo instruments and sterilization equipment used between customers
  - amateur tattoo—often done by adolescents under unclean conditions using straight pins or needles with India ink, carbon, soot, mascara, charcoal, or dirt
- ▲ Associated health risks with tattoos:
  - infection—blood-borne diseases are a concern, as well as infection at the tattoo site itself
  - allergic reactions—allergy may occur to the pigments used in the tattoo
  - granulomas—nodule may form around the particles in the tattoo pigment used
  - kcloid formation—scar tissue that may form as a result of the tattoo

Branding

- ▲ Found in history during the reign of Henry VII (1491–1547)
- ▲ Today, branding is the creation of raised scars on the skin.
- ▲ Accomplished by taking a white-hot piece of metal in a particular shape and pressing it onto a flat area of flesh
- ▲ Healing takes approximately 6 months.
- ▲ Complications:
  - infection—there is great risk of infection as the burn heals and the scar forms
  - skin pigmentation changes
  - development of keloids

TABLE 4–4 • Body Piercing

Location	Jewelry Used	Healing Time	Common Complications
Ampallang	Barbell stud	6–12 months	Keloid formation May interrupt the flow of urine (may need to sit to void) Formation of abscesses, cysts, or boils Ripping and tearing of skin if jewelry gets caught on clothing
Cheek	Labret stud	6–8 weeks	Swelling, infection, gum injury, increased salivation Chipped or broken teeth Speech impairment Aspiration or ingestion of loosened jewelry Difficulty chewing and swallowing Massive systemic infection, septic shock Formation of abscesses, cysts, or boils
Clitoris	Captive bead ring Barbell stud	4–10 weeks	Keloid formation Formation of abscesses, cysts, or boils Ripping and tearing of skin if jewelry gets caught on clothing
Clitoris hood	Captive bead ring Captive stone ring Circular barbell	4–10 weeks	Keloid formation Formation of abscesses, cysts, or boils Ripping and tearing of skin if jewelry gets caught on clothing
Earlobe	Captive bead ring Circular barbell Captive stone ring	4–6 weeks	Keloid formation Formation of abscesses, cysts, or boils Ripping and tearing of skin if jewelry gets caught on clothing
Ear cartilage	Same pieces as an earlobe: larger gauge is used	4–12 months	Keloid formation Formation of abscesses, cysts, or boils Prone to Pseudomonal infections Ripping and tearing of skin if jewelry gets caught on clothing
Earplug	Increases sizes of an object	Gradual enlargement of lobe	Keloid formation Overstretching of skin
Eyebrow	Captive bead ring Captive stone ring Barbell stud	6–8 weeks	Keloid formation Ripping and tearing of skin if jewelry gets caught on clothing Formation of abscesses, cysts, or boils Excess hair growth over piercing area Development of cysts Periorbital cellulitis
Foreskin	Captive bead ring Captive stone ring Circular barbell	6–8 weeks	Formation of abscesses, cysts, or boils Ripping and tearing of skin if jewelry gets caught on clothing
Frenum	Barbell stud	6–8 weeks	Keloid formation Formation of abscesses, cysts, or boils Ripping and tearing of skin if jewelry gets caught on clothing
Hand web	Captive bead ring Captive stone ring Barbell stud	6–12 months	Difficult to heal due to high rate of infection Formation of abscesses, cysts, or boils Ripping and tearing of skin if jewelry gets caught on clothing

TABLE 4-4 • Body Piercing (Continued)

Location	Jewelry Used	Healing Time	Common Complications
Implants	Captive bead ring Captive stone ring Barbell stud Circular barbell Assorted other items, e.g., beads, spikes, coral	2–4 months	Pressure on nerves, blood vessels, and muscles Radiating pain that continues after healing is complete Shifting (when the object moves from its intended place) Rejection by the body's immune system Excess hair growth over implantation area Formation of abscesses, cysts, or boils
Labia majora	Captive bead ring Captive stone ring Circular barbell	6–10 weeks	Keloid formation Formation of abscesses, cysts, or boils Ripping and tearing of skin if jewelry gets caught on clothing
Labia minora	Captive bead ring Captive stone ring Circular barbell	6–10 weeks	Keloid formation Formation of abscesses, cysts, or boils Ripping and tearing of skin if jewelry gets caught on clothing
Lip	Captive bead ring Captive stone ring Barbell stud	2–3 months	Swelling, infection, gingival injury, increased salivation Keloid formation Excess hair growth over pierced area Chipped or broken teeth Speech impairment Aspiration or ingestion of loosened jewelry Massive systemic infection, septic shock Formation of abscesses, cysts, or boils Ripping and tearing of skin if jewelry gets caught on clothing
Nasal septum	Captive bead ring Circular barbell Septum retainer	2–8 months	Formation of abscesses, cysts, or boils Ripping and tearing of skin if jewelry gets caught on clothing

Navel	Captive bead ring
	Captive stone ring
	Circular barbell
		4–12 months	Very slow to heal: redness of area can last for months
			Keloid formation
			Excess hair growth over pierced area
			Very high rate of infection (compared to other piercings) due to:
			  the constant friction rub, movement,
			    bacterial-friendly environment (warm, dark, and moist)
			Formation of abscesses, cysts, or boils
			Ripping and tearing of skin if jewelry gets caught on clothing

Nipples (female)	Captive bead ring
	Captive stone ring
	Circular barbell
		3–6 months	May damage some of the milk-producing ducts
			  May cause problems with future breastfeeding
			    May cause mastitis
			Formation of abscesses, cysts, or boils
			Ripping and tearing of skin if jewelry gets caught on clothing

Nipples (male)	Captive bead ring Captive stone ring Circular barbell	3–6 months	Formation of abscesses, cysts, or boils Ripping and tearing of skin if jewelry gets caught on clothing
Nostril	Captive bead ring Captive stone ring	2–4 months	Keloid formation Formation of abscesses, cysts, or boils Ripping and tearing of skin if jewelry gets caught on clothing

TABLE 4–4 • Body Piercing (Continued)

Location	Jewelry Used	Healing Time	Common Complications
Scrotum	Captive bead ring Captive stone ring Circular barbell	6–8 weeks	Ripping and tearing of skin if jewelry gets caught on clothing
Tongue	Barbell stud	4–6 weeks	Swelling, infection, gingival injury, increased salivation Keloid formation Chipped or broken teeth Speech impairment Aspiration or ingestion of loosened jewelry Difficulty breathing, chewing, and swallowing Prolonged bleeding Massive systemic infection, septic shock Damage to veins and nerves, including neuroma development
Tragus	Captive bead ring Circular barbell Captive stone ring	6–12 months	Formation of abscesses, cysts, or boils
Uvula	Captive bead ring Circular barbell Barbell stud	6–8 weeks	Swelling, infection, injury, increased salivation Speech impairment Aspiration or ingestion of loosened jewelry Difficulty breathing and swallowing Formation of abscesses, cysts, or boils

► USING A TRANSLATOR

How to Get the Most Benefit From a Translator

Communication is a key element in the health care professional's ability to work with, to care for, and to educate patients and their families.

When the patient is a non-English-speaking person, the communication process requires additional patience and concentration on the part of the professional.

For communication to be successful, the ED staff must:

▲ avoid lengthy conversations
▲ utilize short, understandable phrases
▲ use questions that elicit "yes" or "no" answers
▲ be empathetic toward the heightened anxiety and needs of the patient

Key Points That Should Be Remembered

▲ Introduce yourself to the patient and to the translator.
  • You may need to direct the translator to introduce you to the patient.
▲ Verify the translator's ability to interpret appropriately.
  • This can be done by simply stating to the translator, "I would like to see if my English is clear to you" and give some simple directions to follow.
  • If the translator follows your directions and is able to communicate back to you, an assessment can be made as to the translator's ability to interpret accurately.
▲ Let the translator know that his or her knowledge and assistance are appreciated.
▲ Face toward and speak directly to the patient.
  • Refrain from turning to the translator and saying, "Ask her if this hurts."
▲ Be patient, take your time, and progress one sentence at a time.
▲ Resist the tendency to shout.
  • Speak slowly and clearly:
    – emphasize gestures
    – facial expressions
    – tone of voice
▲ Some patients may believe that it is culturally improper for children to know more than adults do and may not speak openly if a child translates for them.
▲ Reproductive issues should be discussed utilizing translator of the same gender.
▲ Verify patient understanding of instructions by asking for return demonstrations or for the patient to repeat given instructions.
▲ By learning a few words of the patient's language, the ED staff member increases his or her rapport with the patient since most patients appreciate the attempt made at communicating on a common ground (Box 4–1).
▲ Document carefully if a translator was used and describe how the patient's understanding of medical care and discharge instructions was determined.

■ Box 4–1: **BASIC SPANISH TRIAGE QUESTIONS**

- Clear communication between health care staff and the patient is essential in the provision of quality care.
- This process of communicating becomes hindered when the patient speaks a language different from that of the ED staff personnel.
- Optimally, the facility should have interpretation services available 24 hours a day.
- Times may arise when there is no interpreter readily available and communication with the patient must occur immediately to ensure the progression of quality patient care.
- Following are some common words and sentences to assist the ED staff when communicating with Spanish-speaking patients.
- The terms are listed in English and Spanish, followed by the pronunciation.

In Spanish, the

G is like **h** before **e** or **i**
J is like **h**
H is always silent
a after a word is the feminine ending

GREETINGS

Hello / Hola (**oh**-*lah*)
Good morning / Buenos días (**bweh**-*nohs* **dee**-*ahs*)
Good afternoon / Buenas tardes (**bweh**-*nahs* **tahr**-*dehs*)
Good evening / Buenas noches (**bweh**-*nahs* **noh**-*chehs*)
How are you? / ¿Cómo está usted? (**koh**-*moh eh*-**stah** *oo*-**stehd**)
Very well, thank you / Muy bien, gracias (*mwee-b'***yehn** **grah**-*s'yahs*)
You're welcome / De nada (*deh* **nah**-*dah*)
Yes / Sí (*see*)
No / No (*noh*)
Maybe / Tal vez (*tahl* **vehs**)
Do you speak English? / ¿Habla usted inglés? (**ah**-*blah oo*-**stehd** *een*-**glehs**)
I speak a little. / Hablo un poquito. (**ah**-*bloh oon poh*-**kee**-*toh*)

Greetings/Registration

Do you understand? / ¿Entiende usted? (*ehn-t'***yehn**-*deh oo*-**stehd**)
I don't understand. / No entiendo. (*noh ehn-t'***yehn**-*doh*)
Repeat, please. / Favor de repetir. (*fah*-**bohr** *deh reh-peh*-**teer**)
My name is ... / Me llamo ... (*meh* **yah**-*moh* ...)
What is your name? / ¿Cómo se llama? (**koh**-*moh seh* **yah**-*mah*)
What is your address? / ¿Cuál es su dirección? (*kwahl ehs soo dee-rek-s'***yohn**) ¿Cuál es su domicilio? (*koo-ahl ehs soo doh-meh*-**sil**-*ee-oh*)
Your telephone number? / ¿Su número de teléfono? (*soo* **noo**-*meh-roh deh teh*-**leh**-*foh-noh*)
How old are you? / ¿Cuántos años tiene? (**kwahn**-*tohs* **ah-n'***yohs* **t'yeh**-*neh*)
What is your date of birth? / ¿Fecha de nacimiento? (**Feh**-*chah deh nah-see-m'***-ehn**-*toh*)
Have you been here before? / ¿Ha estado aquí antes? (*ah eh*-**stah**-*doh ah*-**kee** *ahn*-*tehs*)
Where do you work? / ¿Dónde trabaja? (**Dohn**-*deh trah*-**bah**-*hah*)
Please sign here. / Por favor, firme aquí. (*Pohr fah*-**bohr** *feer*-*meh ah*-**kee**)

(*continued*)

■ Box 4–1: **BASIC SPANISH TRIAGE QUESTIONS (Continued)**

You are giving us permission to treat you here. / Usted nos da permiso de tratarlo(a) aquí. (*Oos*-**tehd** *nohs* **dah** *pehr*-**mee**-*soh deh* trah-**tahr**-*loh[lah] ak*-**kee**)

Where do you come from? / ¿De dónde es? (*deh* **don**-*deh es*) ¿De qué pueblo es? (*deh keh* **pweh**-*blow es*)

TRIAGE QUESTIONS

What happened to you? / ¿Qué le ocurrió? (*keh-lay oh-koo-***rr'yoh**)

When did it happen? / ¿Cuándo ocurrió? (**kwah**-*doh oh-koo-***rr'yoh**)

Has it happened to you before? / ¿Le ha ocurrido antes? (*leh ah oh-koo-***rree**-*doh* **ahn**-*tehs*)

Who is your doctor? / ¿Quién es su doctor/médico? (*k'***yehn** *ehs soo dohk-***tohr/meh**-*dee-koh*)

Where does it hurt? / ¿Dónde le duele? (**dohn**-*deh leh* **dweh**-*leh*)

What medicines do you take? / ¿Cuáles medicinas toma usted? (**kwahl**-*es meh-deh-***see**-*nahs* **toh**-*mah oo-***stehd**)

When was your last normal period? / Cuándo tuvo su última menstruación normal? (**kwan**-*doh* **too**-*boh soo* **ool**-*tee-mah mehns-troo-ahs* '**yohn** *nohr-mahl*)

When was your last tetanus shot? / ¿Cuándo fue la ultima vez que se le inyectó contra el tétano? (**Kwahn**-*doh fweh lah* **ool**-*tee-mah vehs keh seh leh een-yehk-***toh kohn**-*trah ehl teh-***tah**-*noh*)

Did you lose consciousness? / ¿Perdió el conocimiento/ se desmayó? (**Pehr**-*dee-oh ehl koh-noh-see-m'***yehn**-*toh / seh dehs-mah-***yoh**)

For how long? / ¿Por cuánto tiempo? (*pohr* **kwahn**-*toh t'***yehm**-*poh*)

Do you have allergies? / ¿Tiene alergias? (**T'yeh**-*neh ah-***lehr**-*hee-ahs*)

Are you allergic to ... / ¿Tiene alergia contra ... ? (*T'***yeh**-*neh ah-***lehr**-*hee-ah* **con**-*trah ...*)

    foods? / comidas (*koh-***mee**-*dahs*)

    dust? / polvo (**pohl**-*boh*)

    medicines? / medicínas (*meh-dee-***see**-*nahs*)

Do you have ...? / Tiene usted ...? (**T'yeh**-*neh oo-***stehd** *...*)

    asthma? / asma? (**ahs**-*mah?*)

    abdominal pain? / dolor abdomínal? (*doh-***lohr** *ahb-doh-mee* **nahl**)

    backache? / dolor de espalda? (*doh-***lohr** *deh ehs-***pahl**-*dah*)

    chest pain? / dolor en el pecho? (*doh-***lohr** *en ehl* **peh**-*choh*)

    constipation? / estreñimiento? (*esh-treh-n'yee-m'***yehn**-*toh*)

    convulsions? / convulsiones? (*kohn-bool-s'-***ohn**-*ehs*)

    cough? / tos? (*tohs*)

    diabetes? / diabetes? (*dee-ah-***beh**-*tehs*)

    diarrhea? / diarrea? (*dee-ah-***rreh**-*ah*)

    difficulty breathing? / dificultad al respirar? (*dee-fee-kool-***tahd** *ahl rehs-pee-***rahr**)

    ear pain? / dolor de oído? (*doh-***lohr** *deh oh-***ee**-*doh*)

    fever? / fiebre? (**f'yeh**-*breh*)

    headache? / dolor de cabeza? (*doh-***lohr** *deh kah-***beh**-*sah*)

    history of heart problems? / ¿Existe algún problema del corazón en su familia? (*ecks-***is**-*teh al-***goon** *proh-***bleh**-*mah dehl koh-rah-***sohn** *fa-***meel'**-*yah*)

    high blood pressure? / presión alta de la sangre? (*preh-***syohn ahl**-*tah deh lah* **sahn**-*greh*)

    indigestion? / indigestión? (*een-dee-hehs-t'***yohn**)

    lung problems? / problemas en los pulmones? (*proh-***bleh**-*mahs ehn lohs puhl-***moh**-*nehs*)

    nausea? / nausea? (**now**-*oo-seh-ah*)

    neckache? / dolor de cuello? (*doh-***lohr** *deh* **kweh**-*yoh*)

(*continued*)

■ Box 4–1: **BASIC SPANISH TRIAGE QUESTIONS (Continued)**

pain? / dolor? (*doh*-**lohr**)

rash? / erupción de la piel? (eh-roop-**s'yohn** *de lah* **p'yehl**)

sore throat? / dolor de garganta? (*doh*-**lohr** *deh gahr*-**gahn**-*tah*)

stomach ache? / dolor de estómago? (*doh*-**lohr** *deh ehs*-**toh**-*mah-goh*)

vaginal discharge? / una secreción vaginal anormal? (**oo**-*nah seh-kreh*-**s'yohn** *vah-hee*-**nahl** *ah-nohr*-**mahl**)

vomiting? / vómitos? (**voh**-*mee-tos*)

insurance? / ¿plan médico? (*plahn* **meh**-*dee-ko*)

GENERAL INFORMATION

Are you pregnant? / Está embarazada? (*eh*-**stah** *ehm-bah-rah*-**sah**-*dah*)

You will need an x-ray. / Necesita una radiografía. (*neh-seh*-**see**-*tah* **oo**-*nah rah*-d-*'yoh-grah*-**fee**-*ah*)

You will need stitches. / Necesita puntos. (neh-seh-**see**-*tah* **poon**-*tohs*)

Your arm/leg is broken. / Se ha fracturado el brazo/la pierna. (*seh ah frahk-too*-**rah**-*doh ehl* **brah**-*soh/lah* p'**yehr**-*nah*)

It is only a sprain. / Es una torcedura solamente. (*ehs* **oo**-*nah tohr-seh*-**doo**-*rah soh-lah*-**mehn**-*teh*)

I am calling a specialist to see you. / Voy a llamar a un especialista para que lo/la vea. (*voy ah yah*-**mahr** *ah oon eh-speh-s'yah*-**lee**-*stah pah-rah keh loh[lah]* **veh**-*ah*)

You will need an operation. / Necesita una operación (cirugia). (*neh-seh*-**see**-*tah* **oo**-*nah oh-peh-rah*-**s'yohn** [*see-roo*-**hee**-*ah*])

I am going to give you an injection. / Le voy a poner una inyección. (*leh voy ah poh*-**nehr** **oo**-*nah een-yehk*-**s'yohn**)

You will have to wait 30 minutes. / Tendrá que esperar por lo menos treinta minutos. (*Tehn*-**drah** *keh ehs-peh*-**rahr** *pohr loh* **meh**-*nohs* **train**-*tah mee-noo*-*tohs*)

I am going to place an intravenous needle in your arm. / Le voy a poner una aguja intravenosa en el brazo. (*le boy a poh*-**nehr** **oo**-*nah ah-goo*-*hah een-trah-veh*-**noh**-*sah ehn ehl* **brah**-*soh*)

Have this prescription filled. / Haga preparar esta receta. (**ah**-*gah preh-pah*-**rahr** **eh**-*stah reh-seh*-*tah*)

Who should we call to come get you? / A quién podemos llamar para que lo/la lleve a su casa? (*ah* k'**yehn**-*an poh*-**day**-*mos yah*-**mahr** *pah-rah kay lo* **yeh**-*veh ah soo* **kah**-*sah*)

1 one / uno (**oo**-*noh*)
2 two / dos (*dohs*)
3 three / tres (*trehs*)
4 four / cuatro (**koo-ah**-*troh*)
5 five / cinco (**seen**-*koh*)
6 six / seis (*seh-ees*)
7 seven / siete (*see*-**eh**-*teh*)
8 eight / ocho (**oh**-*choh*)
9 nine / nueve (*new*-**eh**-*veh*)
10 ten / diez (*dee*-**ehs**)
20 twenty / veinte (**beh**-*een-teh*)
30 thirty / treinta (**treh**-*een-tah*)
40 forty / cuarenta (*koo-ah*-**rehn**-*tah*)
50 fifty / cincuenta (*seen*-**kwen**-*tah*)
60 sixty / sesenta (*seh*-**sehn**-*tah*)
70 seventy / setenta (*seh*-**tehn**-*tah*)
80 eighty / ochenta (*oh*-**chehn**-*tah*)

(continued)

■ Box 4–1: **BASIC SPANISH TRIAGE QUESTIONS (Continued)**

90 ninety / noventa (*noh-***behn**-*tah*)
100 one hundred / cien (*see-***ehn**)
January / Enero (*Eh-***neh**-*roh*)
February / Febrero (*Feh-***breh**-*roh*)
March / Marzo (**Mahr**-*soh*)
April / Abril (*Ah-***breel**)
May / Mayo (**Mah**-*yoh*)
June / Junio (**Hoo**-*nee-oh*)
July / Julio (**Hoo**-*lee-oh*)
August / Agosto (*Ah-***gohs**-*toh*)
September / Septiembre (*Sehp-tee-***ehm**-*breh*)
October / Octubre (*Ohk-***too**-*breh*)
November / Noviembre (*Noh-bee-***ehm**-*breh*)
December / Diciembre (*Dee-see-***ehm**-*breh*)

► TELEPHONE TRIAGE

Telephone triage has become an essential part of health care in our society and around the world. Emergency departments, urgent care centers, and physicians' offices receive telephone inquiries from a wide range of patients in the surrounding community and from distant places. For telephone triage to be practiced safely and effectively, an *organized system must be in place*. Without a developed program to follow, the practice of giving advice over a telephone is unsafe in every imaginable way.

The goal of telephone triage is similar to that of face-to-face triage—determining the level of care needed by the patient and assigning an acuity level. On the telephone, however, a strong knowledge background, clinical expertise, established protocols, excellent listening and communication skills, and a sense of intuition guide the nurse. The nurse no longer has the additional senses (touch, smell, and sight) to assist in the assessment process and must rely solely on what the caller says and does not say.

In concert with or in addition to the qualifications listed earlier in the book for ED triage, a telephone triage nurse should have:

▲ a solid history of "hands-on" experience in the specialty area in which telephone triage will be performed
▲ demonstrated comfort with working independently and autonomously with precision critical-thinking skills
▲ established tools, including policies, protocols, guidelines, and algorithms
▲ expertise in patient assessment skills; ability to identify potentially or actual life-threatening situations
▲ solid comfort in the ability to assign acuity to each telephone patient assessment
▲ precision documentation skills
▲ high morale and work ethics
▲ certification in Telephone Nursing Practice
  • must have current U.S. or Canadian licensure
  • minimum of 2 years' experience in telephone nursing practice

Protocols are more in-depth than most face-to-face triage protocols, and a sample is included (Box 4–2). The nurse performs an assessment and recommends treatment and when it is necessary—the level of care at the safest interval (immediately vs. 24 hours from now).

■ Box 4–2: SAMPLE PROTOCOL FOR TELEPHONE TRIAGE: ABDOMINAL PAIN

A. Obtain and record telephone triage assessment that includes:
  1. Description of pain
    • **P**rovoking factors (what makes it worse/better?)
    • **Q**uality of pain
    • **R**egion/radiation
    • **S**everity of pain
    • **T**ime (onset, duration)
    • **T**reatment (what has the patient already tried?)
  2. Associated symptoms and behavior
    • known trauma
    • fever

(continued)

■ Box 4–2: **SAMPLE PROTOCOL FOR TELEPHONE TRIAGE: ABDOMINAL PAIN** (**Continued**)

- irritability
- poor appetite
- chest pain
- difficulty walking
- gravid history
- penile discharge
- LNMP
- last bowel movement
- nausea/vomiting/diarrhea
- difficulty breathing
- urinary symptoms
  - frequency
  - hematuria
  - burning
- vaginal discharge or unusual bleeding
- change in activity level
- possible ingestion of chemical, plants, medications, etc.

B. Risk factors that increase the acuity of abdominal pain include:
- history of abdominal surgery
- diabetes
- chronic/congenital illness
- irregular menses in sexually active female
- history of abdominal injury

C. See immediately

The triage nurse should advise the use of an ambulance when the patient's current status is life-threatening, may deteriorate en route to hospital, or anxiety level is too high to safely drive patient to closest ED.

- recent abdominal trauma
- pain is localized to lower abdomen (either side) for more than 1 to 2 hours
- inconsolable child or constant crying for more than 2 hours
- marked change in activity level for more than 1 hour:
  - refuses to walk
  - painful to climb stairs
  - lying with knees drawn up to chest
  - walks bent over, holding abdomen
- severe pain if patient or child jumps on one foot
- rapidly increasing pain
- pain in scrotum or testicle
- grossly bloody bowel movements or jelly-like stools
- vomiting blood or bile on more than one occasion
- possibility of ingestion or poisoning (plant, chemical, medicine, foreign body)
- unusually heavy vaginal bleeding or chance of pregnancy
- patient sounds very sick or weak to the triage nurse

(continued)

■ Box 4–2: **SAMPLE PROTOCOL FOR TELEPHONE TRIAGE: ABDOMINAL PAIN (Continued)**

D. See within 12 to 24 hours if:
  • pain lasts longer than 24 hours
  • urinary symptoms are present (frequency, burning, hematuria, etc.)
  • severe nausea/vomiting/diarrhea with risk of dehydration
  • fever over 101°F (38.3°C), cough, weakness, sore throat
  • persistent nausea/vomiting/diarrhea unresponsive to home care
  • vaginal or urethral discharge
  • weight loss
E. Home care advice
  • Encourage lying down and resting.
  • Have vomiting pan handy.
  • Suggest sitting on toilet and trying to pass a bowel movement.
  • Offer clear liquids only and slowly progress to a bland diet for 12 to 24 hours.
    • may use rehydrating fluid solution for infants and small children
    • recommend taking any medications that may cause stomach upset with food
F. Call back if:
  • pain worsens, develops new symptoms, or if symptoms change
  • severe pain present after 1 hour of rest
  • constant pain persisting for longer than 2 hours
  • intermittent pain for longer than 24 hours
  • pain worsens with heat or activity
  • urine, stool, or emesis contains blood
  • fever
  • persistent vomiting or diarrhea
  • increased concern or anxiety

EMERGENCY MEDICAL TREATMENT AND ACTIVE LABOR ACT (EMTALA)

▲ In 1986, the government passed the Consolidated Omnibus Budget Reconciliation Act (COBRA) law to address the problem of "patient dumping"—the denial of care or transfer of patients based on their inability to pay for their care.

▲ The law has been updated regularly and currently states that a hospital that received Medicare benefits are required to:

1. Provide a *medical screening exam* to all patients who present upon the hospital premises
   - The hospital is required to accept and evaluate any patient on its premises who presents for a non-scheduled visit and seeks care, regardless of ability to pay.
   - Triage assessment does not constitute a medical screening exam.
   - *Hospital premises* includes:
     - hospital-owned and -operated ambulances and off-campus locations billing under the same Medicare provider number
     - areas, facilities, or services contained in the hospital's operating certificate (hospital-owned clinics, MD practices, etc.)

2. Provide stabilizing care
   - Very strict interpretation of the word "stable"
     - Patients must not be at risk of deterioration from, during, or following transfer or discharge.
   - A pregnant woman having contractions is not *legally stable* until the baby and placenta are delivered.
     - This applies to in-house patients as well as ED patients.

3. May NOT transfer patients who are potentially unstable if the hospital has the capabilities on site and the physical capacity to treat the patient
   - Patients may only be transferred for medical necessity, not physician convenience or practice preferences.
   - Under EMTALA, a transfer is defined as any time the patient leaves the hospital campus, including discharge, unless AMA or deceased.

4. Maintain an on-call system to be able to provide services required to stabilize patients
   - The on-call list must include every specialty service privileged at the hospital (unless too few physicians exist in a specialty to provide coverage on call—there are special rules that will apply in those situations).
   - The on-call list must be posted in a conspicuous location in the ED and include the name of an individual responsible for call, at any given time.
   - This list must be accurately maintained for 5 years.
   - On-call physicians MUST respond to the hospital and render evaluation and care in the hospital.
     - It is NOT permissible to send patients to a specialist's office for definitive care.
   - If the on-call physician refuses to come in to evaluate a patient, an EMTALA violation will occur against the physician as well as the hospital.

5. Provide patients with transfers that are medically necessitated. This process must include:
   - Physician certification at the time of transfer, which states the risks of transfer are outweighed by the reasonably anticipated benefits. Specific individual risks and benefits must be listed and the record must support them.

OR

   - Written request by the patient for a transfer, without suggestion or pressure of the caring hospital or physician to induce such a request by the patient

- Advanced acceptance by the destination hospital, which is well documented in the patient's record
- Written consent for the transfer, signed by the patient
- Transfer by appropriate medical transfer vehicle; private passenger vehicles are not permitted unless ambulance transport has been refused in writing.
- Medical orders for appropriate attendant personnel during transport, who have the skill and expertise to provide the level of care required for the patient
- Medical orders for appropriate life support equipment; assurance that transport vehicle is appropriately equipped to provide the level of care needed by the patient.
- Copies of the medical records, tests, and x-rays must be sent with the patient, unless the delay for records could jeopardize the patient. If a patient is sent without copies of his or her records, then the records must be transported to the receiving hospital as soon as completed and on a STAT basis.
6. Accepts requests for incoming transfer if the hospital has the specialized capabilities needed by the patient, and the transferring hospital is relatively less able to care for the patient (Frew, 2002).

Figure 4–3 illustrates a sample *consent to transfer* form that complies with EMTALA rules and regulations.

EMTALA Transfer Consent

STEP 1: DEMOGRAPHIC, MEDICAL SCREEN, and STABILIZATION

Patient's Name _____ Patient's Attending MD _____

Medical Record # _____ Transferring Facility _____

A Medical Screening Evaluation was performed on this patient by: _____ MD

    ❏ Emergency Medical Condition Exists

    ❏ *No* Emergency Medical Condition Exists

    ❏ Unable to complete the medical screening evaluation

Stabilization status:

    ❏ The patient has been stabilized within reasonable medical probability and no deterioration of patient's condition is expected to occur during transfer to receiving facility.

    ❏ The patient's condition has been stabilized the best possible, given the need for emergent transfer.

STEP 2: CONSENT to TRANSFER

Potential Risks and Benefits of Transfer discussed with patient/family:

* This patient and/or legal representative acting on behalf of the patient has been informed of the risks and benefits involved in this transfer and chooses to: ❏ consent ❏ request ❏ refuse

* If patient/representative refuses, list the reasons _____

* Authorized signature and relationship to patient: _____

* If patient/representative unable to sign, the physician must sign here: _____

STEP 3: TRANSFER INFORMATION

* Reason for transfer _____

* Name of receiving facility _____

* **Name of physician accepting** patient transfer _____

* Mode of transportation: ❏ ground transport   ❏ air transport (helicopter or fixed wing)

* Check one: ❏ Medical records have been copied and sent with patient being transferred.

        ❏ Medical records not available at this time, and will be faxed or delivered as soon as available.

        ** You must document what date and time this was accomplished as well as verifying with the receiving facility that they have received the medical records.

STEP 4: TRANSFER PHYSICIAN CERTIFICATION

I certify that I have answered the above questions to the best of my knowledge. Based on the reasonable risk and benefits to the patient, as noted above, and based on the information available to me at the time of this patient's transfer, the medical benefits reasonably expected from the treatment of this patient at another facility outweigh the increased risks, if any, to this patient's (and/or her fetus's) health condition from transfer.

* Physician's signature: _____

* Print name: _____ Date and Time: _____

If name of physician completing this form is different from the certifying physician, then sign here: _____MD

(Original copy of this form goes to accepting facility, copy stays with sending facility.)

Figure 4–3. EMTALA Transfer Consent Form.

CE Tests

CE Enrollment Form

A Quick Reference to Triage — Part I — Triage Process

A. Registration Information:

Last name _____ First name _____ MI _____

Address _____

City _____ State _____ Zip _____

Telephone _____ Fax _____ email _____

Registration Deadline: (APRIL 30, 2005)
Contact Hours: 2
Fee: $14.95

B. Test Answers: Darken one for your answer to each question.

	A	B	C	D			A	B	C	D
1.	❏	❏	❏	❏		6.	❏	❏	❏	❏
2.	❏	❏	❏	❏		7.	❏	❏	❏	❏
3.	❏	❏	❏	❏		8.	❏	❏	❏	❏
4.	❏	❏	❏	❏		9.	❏	❏	❏	❏
5.	❏	❏	❏	❏		10.	❏	❏	❏	❏

C. Evaluation*

		A	B
1. Did this CE activity's learning objectives relate to its general purpose?		❏ yes	❏ no
2. Was the journal home study format an effective way to present the material?		❏ yes	❏ no
3. Was the content relevant to your nursing practice?		❏ yes	❏ no

4. How long did it take you to complete this CE activity?_____hours_____minutes
5. Suggestion for future topics_____

D. Two Easy Ways to Pay:

❏ Check or money order enclosed
(Payable to Lippincott Williams & Wilkins)
Charge my ❏ Mastercard ❏ Visa ❏ American Express
Card #_____Exp. Date _____
Signature_____

*In accordance with the Iowa Board of Nursing Administrative rules governing grievances, a copy of your evaluation activity may be submitted directly to the Iowa Board of Nursing.

CE Enrollment Form

A Quick Reference to Triage — Part I — Triage Process

❏ LPN   ❏ RN   ❏ CNS   ❏ NP   ❏ CRNA   ❏ CNM   ❏ other

Job Title _____ Specialty _____

Type of Facility _____

Are you certified?   ❏ yes   ❏ no

Certified by _____

State of License (1) _____ License # _____

State of License (2) _____ License # _____

Social Security # _____

❏ From time to time we make our mailing list available to outside organizations to announce special offers. Please check here if you do not wish us to release your name and address.

CE Test

A Quick Reference to Triage
Part I – Triage Process

Instructions:

- Read **Part** I on page **1**.
- Take the test, recording your answers in the test answers section (Section B) of the CE enrollment form. Each question has only one correct answer.
- Complete registration information (Section A) and course evaluation (Section C).
- Mail completed test with registration fee to: Lippincott Williams & Wilkins, CE Depart., 345 Hudson Street, New York, NY 10014.
- Within 3–4 weeks after your CE enrollment form is received, you will be notified of your test results.
- If you pass, you will receive a certificate of earned contact hours and answer key. If you fail, you have the option of taking the test again at no additional cost.
- A passing score for this test is **7** correct answers.
- Need CE STAT? Call 800-833-6525 x331 or x332 for rush service options.
- Questions? Contact Lippincott, Williams & Wilkins: (212) 886-1331 or (212) 886-1332.

Registration Deadline: APRIL 30, 2005.

Provider Accreditation:

This Continuing Nursing Education (CNE) activity for **2** contact hours is provided by Lippincott Williams & Wilkins, which is accredited as a provider of continuing education in nursing by the American Nurses Credentialing Center's Commission on Accreditation and by the American Association of Critical-Care Nurses (AACN 9722, CERP Category A). This activity is also provider approved by the California Board of Registered Nursing, Provider Number CEP 11749, for **2** contact hours. LWW is also an approved provider of CNE in Alabama, Florida, and Iowa and holds the following provider numbers: AL #ABNP0114, FL #FBN2454, IA #75. All of its home study activities are classified for Texas nursing continuing education requirements as Type I.

Your certificate is valid in all states. This means that your certificate of earned contact hours is valid no matter where you live.

Payment and Discounts:

- The registration fee for this test is $14.95.
- If you take two or more tests in this book and send in your CE enrollment forms together, you may deduct $1.00 from the price of each test.
- We offer special discounts for as few as six tests and institutional bulk discounts for multiple tests. Call (800) 346-7844, ext. 1286 for more information.

General Purpose: To provide registered professional nurses with an overview of the triage process.

Objectives: After reading this chapter and taking this test you will be able to:

1. Discuss how to perform a basic triage assessment.
2. Describe how to determine a patient's acuity status.

1. **Which of these statements regarding triage evaluation is correct?**
   a. The triage nurse should be able to interview and perform a physical assessment of the patient within 4–5 minutes.
   b. A complete head-to-toe assessment by the triage nurse is necessary when a patient presents with a potentially life-threatening illness.
   c. Patients should register with hospital personnel prior to receiving a triage evaluation by a nurse.
   d. Patients who arrive with a nonurgent condition should receive a triage evaluation within 30 minutes.

2. **Greg Johnson, a 37-year-old male, presents to the triage area of the emergency department. Which of the following statements should the triage nurse make to the patient *first*?**
   a. "Mr. Johnson, I need you to spell your first and last name."
   b. "Please describe why you came to the emergency department."
   c. "My name is Anne Smith and I am a registered nurse who will be performing your initial assessment."
   d. "I am going to be asking you a series of questions about your medical history in order to determine what type of care you will require."

3. **When assessing orthostatic vital signs of a patient in order to assign acuity level in triage, the *most important* for you to do is**
   a. obtain the patient's vital signs with the patient positioned in the supine (if available), sitting, and standing positions.
   b. assess the patient's radial and apical rates simultaneously with a colleague and compare the rates.
   c. check the amplitude of the patient's arterial pulse during inspiration while measuring the blood pressure.
   d. check for jugular pulsation while pressing into the patient's right upper abdominal quadrant for 30 seconds.

4. **A patient with abdominal pain is *most likely* to use which of these words to describe the pain?**
   a. squeezing, pressure, cramping, dull, and/or deep
   b. burning, shooting, tingling, and/or radiating
   c. aching, throbbing, sore, and/or twinge
   d. smarting, numb, stinging, and/or tender

5. **Using the five-level acuity system, a 30-year-old female patient who has burning with urination and a vaginal discharge for several days would be classified as**
   a. level 2, emergent.
   b. level 3, urgent.
   c. level 4, semi-urgent.
   d. level 5, routine.

6. **A male patient is released from the ED with a diagnosis of influenza. The following day he returns to the ED reporting no change in his condition. When triaging this patient, it would be important for you to know that**
   a. patients who return to the ED within 72 hours are known to be high-risk.
   b. patients most commonly return to the ED because of drug-seeking behavior.
   c. patients most commonly return to the ED because the discharge instructions were not understood.
   d. patients who return to the ED within 24 hours do not require a complete medical screening exam.

7. **When assessing a patient for an allergy to latex, you should ask the patient if**
   a. malignant hyperthermia ever developed following anesthesia.
   b. a red discoloration of the skin has ever developed after taking acetaminophen.
   c. swelling of the lips or shortness of breath has ever developed after eating peanuts.
   d. burning, swelling, or hives has ever occurred after the patient has blown up a balloon.

8. **A 14-year-old female patient is brought to the emergency department by a parent who reports that her daughter is acting "strange." When obtaining a brief triage history, you should ask**
   a. the parent if the patient recently received the Lyme vaccine.
   b. the patient the date of her last normal menstrual period (LNMP).
   c. the patient if she has engaged in sexual intercourse within the past 24 hours.
   d. the parent if there is a family history of depression, bipolar disorder, or schizophrenia.

9. **A 16-year-old patient's mother informs you that she thinks her son has taken an unknown quantity of a tricyclic antidepressant. Using the five-level acuity system, the patient should be treated and reassessed within**
   a. 5–15 minutes.
   b. 20–45 minutes.
   c. 45–60 minutes.
   d. 1–2 hours.

10. **It would indicate correct use of the five-level acuity system if a patient with**
    a. severe emotional distress is treated immediately.
    b. alcohol or drug intoxication is treated within 5–15 minutes.
    c. noncardiac chest pain is treated within 15–45 minutes.
    d. an earache is treated within four hours.

CE Enrollment Form

A Quick Reference to Triage — Part II — Triage Guidelines

A. Registration Information:

Last name _____ First name _____ MI _____

Address _____

City _____ State _____ Zip _____

Telephone _____ Fax _____ email _____

Registration Deadline: (APRIL 30, 2005)
Contact Hours: 4
Fee: $27.00

B. Test Answers: Darken one for your answer to each question.

	A	B	C	D		A	B	C	D		A	B	C	D
1.	❒	❒	❒	❒	11.	❒	❒	❒	❒	21.	❒	❒	❒	❒
2.	❒	❒	❒	❒	12.	❒	❒	❒	❒	22.	❒	❒	❒	❒
3.	❒	❒	❒	❒	13	❒	❒	❒	❒	23.	❒	❒	❒	❒
4.	❒	❒	❒	❒	14.	❒	❒	❒	❒	24.	❒	❒	❒	❒
5.	❒	❒	❒	❒	15.	❒	❒	❒	❒	25.	❒	❒	❒	❒
6.	❒	❒	❒	❒	16.	❒	❒	❒	❒	26.	❒	❒	❒	❒
7.	❒	❒	❒	❒	17.	❒	❒	❒	❒	27.	❒	❒	❒	❒
8.	❒	❒	❒	❒	18.	❒	❒	❒	❒	28.	❒	❒	❒	❒
9.	❒	❒	❒	❒	19.	❒	❒	❒	❒	29.	❒	❒	❒	❒
10.	❒	❒	❒	❒	20.	❒	❒	❒	❒	30.	❒	❒	❒	❒

C. Evaluation*

	A	B
1. Did this CE activity's learning objectives relate to its general purpose?	❒ yes	❒ no
2. Was the home study format an effective way to present the material?	❒ yes	❒ no
3. Was the content relevant to your nursing practice?	❒ yes	❒ no

4. How long did it take you to complete this CE activity?_____hours_____minutes
5. Suggestion for future topics_____

D. Two Easy Ways to Pay:

❒ Check or money order enclosed
(Payable to Lippincott Williams & Wilkins)
Charge my ❒ Mastercard ❒ Visa ❒ American Express
Card #_____ Exp. Date_____
Signature_____

*In accordance with the Iowa Board of Nursing Administrative rules governing grievances, a copy of your evaluation activity may be submitted directly to the Iowa Board of Nursing.

CE Enrollment Form

A Quick Reference to Triage — Part II — Triage Guidelines

❏ LPN   ❏ RN   ❏ CNS   ❏ NP   ❏ CRNA   ❏ CNM   ❏ other

Job Title _____ Specialty _____

Type of Facility _____

Are you certified?   ❏ yes   ❏ no

Certified by _____

State of License (1) _____ License # _____

State of License (2) _____ License # _____

Social Security # _____

❏ From time to time we make our mailing list available to outside organizations to announce special offers. Please check here if you do not wish us to release your name and address.

CE Test

A Quick Reference to Triage
Part II – Triage Guidelines

Instructions:

- Read **Part II** on page **21.**
- Take the test, recording your answers in the test answers section (Section B) of the CE enrollment form. Each question has only one correct answer.
- Complete registration information (Section A) and course evaluation (Section C).
- Mail completed test with registration fee to: Lippincott Williams & Wilkins, CE Depart., 345 Hudson Street, New York, NY 10014.
- Within 3–4 weeks after your CE enrollment form is received, you will be notified of your test results.
- If you pass, you will receive a certificate of earned contact hours and answer key. If you fail, you have the option of taking the test again at no additional cost.
- A passing score for this test is **23** correct answers.
- Need CE STAT? Call 800-833-6525 x331 or x332 for rush service options.
- Questions? Contact Lippincott Williams & Wilkins: (212) 886-1331 or (212) 886-1332.

Registration Deadline: APRIL 30, 2005.

Provider Accreditation:

This Continuing Nursing Education (CNE) activity for **4** contact hours is provided by Lippincott Williams & Wilkins, which is accredited as a provider of continuing education in nursing by the American Nurses Credentialing Center's Commission on Accreditation and by the American Association of Critical-Care Nurses (AACN 9722, CERP Category A). This activity is also provider approved by the California Board of Registered Nursing, Provider Number CEP 11749, for **4** contact hours. LWW is also an approved provider of CNE in Alabama, Florida, and Iowa and holds the following provider numbers: AL #ABNP0114, FL #FBN2454, IA #75. All of its home study activities are classified for Texas nursing continuing education requirements as Type I.

Your certificate is valid in all states. This means that your certificate of earned contact hours is valid no matter where you live.

Payment and Discounts:

- The registration fee for this test is $27.00.
- If you take two or more tests in this book and send in your CE enrollment forms together, you may deduct $1.00 from the price of each test.
- We offer special discounts for as few as six tests and institutional bulk discounts for multiple tests. Call (800) 346-7844; ext. 1286 for more information.

General Purpose: To present registered professional nurses with detailed assessment information for evaluating clinical situations.

Objectives: After reading this chapter and taking this test, you will be able to:

1. Discuss concepts, definitions, and principles helpful in triaging the types of situations described.
2. Describe key assessment tools or guidelines to use when assessing patients.
3. Outline interventions for patients undergoing triage.

1. **In the PQRSTT mnemonic often used to evaluate pain, the "P" refers to**
   a. persistence.
   b. provoking factors.
   c. palpability.
   d. perception.

2. **A patient over the age of 50 who presents with abdominal pain should receive immediate care when which of the following is also present?**
   a. a pulse rate of 92
   b. a pulse rate of 64
   c. a blood pressure of 90/64
   d. a blood pressure of 144/96

3. **Abdominal pain radiating to the right shoulder is a classic symptom of**
   a. cholelithiasis.
   b. abdominal aortic aneurysm.
   c. pancreatitis.
   d. renal calculi.

4. **Which of the following patients meets burn center transfer criteria?**
   a. a 40-year-old man with second- and third-degree burns over 18% of his body
   b. a 35-year-old man with second- and third-degree burns on his feet
   c. an 8-year-old girl with second- and third-degree burns over 9% of her body
   d. a 75-year-old man with second- and third-degree burns over 9% of his body

5. **Basic initial wound care when a minor burn is still warm includes**
   a. applying ice to cool the wound.
   b. applying a warm sterile compress to maintain circulation.
   c. applying a cool, moist sterile compress.
   d. keeping the wound open to air.

6. **Which of the following carboxyhemoglobin saturation levels is likely to cause tachycardia and tachypnea?**
   a. 15%   b. 25%   c. 35%   d. 45%

7. **Alkaline burns require copious lavage with water or saline for**
   a. 15 minutes.   b. 30 minutes.   c. 30 minutes to 1 hour.   d. 1 to 2 hours.

8. **Chest pain that worsens when the patient lies on his left side is a classic symptom of**
   a. pericarditis.   b. angina.   c. GERD.   d. pulmonary embolism.

9. **Respiratory isolation is indicated for a patient who presents with difficulty breathing as well as**
   a. crackles and ashen skin.
   b. night sweats and debilitating fatigue.
   c. stridor and pallor.
   d. cyanosis and wheezing.

10. A dark purple bruise is likely to have been inflicted
    a. in the last 1 to 2 hours.   c. 1 to 4 days ago.
    b. over the last 24 hours.   d. 5 to 7 days ago.

11. Vomiting in patients with altered glucose metabolism is a sign of
    a. hypoglycemia.   c. insulin shock.
    b. diabetic ketoacidosis.   d. hyperglycemic hyperosmolar nonketotic coma.

12. Painless loss of vision in one eye is a sign of
    a. central retinal artery occlusion.   c. periorbital cellulitis.
    b. glaucoma.   d. a detached retina.

13. To increase the chances of successful reimplantation of an avulsed tooth, place the tooth in
    a. warm tap water.   b. milk.   c. vinegar.   d. hydrogen peroxide.

14. Which of the following is a sign of pelvic inflammatory disease?
    a. painful genital lesions   b. cellulitis   c. abdominal pain   d. perineal itch

15. Which of the following is most likely to be asymptomatic?
    a. chlamydia trachomatis   c. bacterial vaginosis
    b. trichomonas vaginalis   d. candida albicans

16. A severe headache with facial swelling is characteristic of
    a. meningitis.   c. cerebellar hemorrhage.
    b. cluster headaches.   d. migraine headaches.

17. When assessing cold-induced injuries, it is important to remember that
    a. tissue loss is inevitable.
    b. the initial appearance of the injury is a good predictor of the outcome.
    c. frostbite always involves bone.
    d. ice crystals will form in extracellular spaces if tissue temperature drops below 59°F.

18. The incubation period for chlamydia is
    a. 4–14 days.
    b. entire period of the infection.
    c. many weeks prior to the onset of the first symptom.
    d. unknown.

19. Which of the following communicable diseases can be transmitted from person to person?
    a. hand, foot, and mouth disease   c. Rocky Mountain spotted fever
    b. Legionnaire's disease   d. botulism

20. If a psychiatric patient is considered a flight risk, which of the following is recommended?
    a. placing him in isolation
    b. removing his clothes
    c. restraining him
    d. explaining that he must stay until he is evaluated by a physician

21. **All of the following are signs of alcohol withdrawal *except***
    a. hypotension.　　b. dehydration.　　c. depression.　　d. anorexia.

22. **Sexual promiscuity is a classic manifestation of**
    a. obsessive-compulsive disorder.　　c. schizophrenia.
    b. borderline personality disorder.　　d. bipolar disorder.

23. **Painless vaginal bleeding in the third trimester of pregnancy is a sign of**
    a. eclampsia.　　　　　　c. premature rupture of membranes.
    b. abruptio placenta.　　d. placenta previa.

24. **A fracture of the growth plate in children is called a**
    a. LeFort fracture.　　　　c. Salter-Harris fracture.
    b. greenstick fracture.　　d. prelongitudinal fracture.

25. **An elevated, solid lesion larger than 2 cm in diameter is a**
    a. papule.　　b. plaque.　　c. nodule.　　d. tumor.

26. **Reddish, purplish spots that do not blanch are**
    a. spider angiomas.　　b. venous stars.　　c. purpura.　　d. telangiectasia.

27. **Of the following, the biological agent-induced disease with the lowest mortality rate is**
    a. tularemia.　　b. botulism.　　c. anthrax.　　d. viral hemorrhagic fevers.

28. **Presence of a radial pulse in a trauma patient indicates that the patient's systolic blood pressure is at least**
    a. 60 mm Hg.　　b. 70 mm Hg.　　c. 80 mm Hg.　　d. 90 mm Hg.

29. **When caring for pediatric trauma patients, it is important to remember that**
    a. the flexibility of children's skeletons helps prevent damage to internal organs.
    b. children can lose up to 25% of their blood volume before their blood pressure decreases.
    c. children need relatively fewer calories due to their lower metabolic rate.
    d. head injuries are the leading cause of trauma-related death in children.

30. **Which of the following is considered a potentially infectious material?**
    a. urine　　b. vomitus　　c. tears　　d. amniotic fluid

CE Enrollment Form

A Quick Reference to Triage — Part III — Pearls of Triage Wisdom

A. Registration Information:

Last name _____ First name _____ MI _____

Address _____

City _____ State _____ Zip _____

Telephone _____ Fax _____ email _____

Registration Deadline: (APRIL 30, 2005)
Contact Hours: 2
Fee: $14.95

B. Test Answers: Darken one for your answer to each question.

	A	B	C	D			A	B	C	D
1.	❐	❐	❐	❐		6.	❐	❐	❐	❐
2.	❐	❐	❐	❐		7.	❐	❐	❐	❐
3.	❐	❐	❐	❐		8.	❐	❐	❐	❐
4.	❐	❐	❐	❐		9.	❐	❐	❐	❐
5.	❐	❐	❐	❐		10.	❐	❐	❐	❐

C. Evaluation*

	A	B
1. Did this CE activity's learning objectives relate to its general purpose?	❐ yes	❐ no
2. Was the home study format an effective way to present the material?	❐ yes	❐ no
3. Was the content relevant to your nursing practice?	❐ yes	❐ no

4. How long did it take you to complete this CE activity?_____hours_____minutes
5. Suggestion for future topics_____

D. Two Easy Ways to Pay:

❐ Check or money order enclosed
(Payable to Lippincott Williams & Wilkins)
Charge my ❐ Mastercard ❐ Visa ❐ American Express
Card #_____Exp. Date_____
Signature_____

*In accordance with the Iowa Board of Nursing Administrative rules governing grievances, a copy of your evaluation activity may be submitted directly to the Iowa Board of Nursing.

CE Enrollment Form

A Quick Reference to Triage — Part III — Pearls of Triage Wisdom

❏ LPN   ❏ RN   ❏ CNS   ❏ NP   ❏ CRNA   ❏ CNM   ❏ other

Job Title _____ Specialty _____

Type of Facility _____

Are you certified?   ❏ yes   ❏ no

Certified by _____

State of License (1) _____ License # _____

State of License (2) _____ License # _____

Social Security # _____

❏ From time to time we make our mailing list available to outside organizations to announce special offers. Please check here if you do not wish us to release your name and address.

CE Test

A Quick Reference to Triage
Part III – Pearls of Triage Wisdom

Instructions:

- Read **Part III** on page **189.**
- Take the test, recording your answers in the test answers section (Section B) of the CE enrollment form. Each question has only one correct answer.
- Complete registration information (Section A) and course evaluation (Section C).
- Mail completed test with registration fee to: Lippincott Williams & Wilkins, CE Depart, 345 Hudson Street, New York, NY 10014.
- Within 3–4 weeks after your CE enrollment form is received, you will be notified of your test results.
- If you pass, you will receive a certificate of earned contact hours and answer key. If you fail, you have the option of taking the test again at no additional cost.
- A passing score for this test is **7** correct answers.
- Need CE STAT? Call 800-833-6525 x331 or x332 for rush service options.
- Questions? Contact Lippincott Williams & Wilkins: (212) 886-1331 or (212) 886-1332.

Registration Deadline: APRIL 30, 2005.

Provider Accreditation:

This Continuing Nursing Education (CNE) activity for **2** contact hours is provided by Lippincott Williams & Wilkins, which is accredited as a provider of continuing education in nursing by the American Nurses Credentialing Center's Commission on Accreditation and by the American Association of Critical-Care Nurses (AACN 9722, CERP Category A). This activity is also provider approved by the California Board of Registered Nursing, Provider Number CEP 11749, for **2** contact hours. LWW is also an approved provider of CNE in Alabama, Florida, and Iowa and holds the following provider numbers: AL #ABNP0114, FL #FBN2454, IA #75. All of its home study activities are classified for Texas nursing continuing education requirements as Type I.

Your certificate is valid in all states. This means that your certificate of earned contact hours is valid no matter where you live.

Payment and Discounts:

- The registration fee for this test is $14.95.
- If you take two or more tests in this book and send in your CE enrollment forms together, you may deduct $1.00 from the price of each test.
- We offer special discounts for as few as six tests and institutional bulk discounts for multiple tests. Call (800) 346-7844, ext. 1286 for more information.

General Purpose: To provide registered professional nurses with information on triage assessment protocols for geriatric, psychiatric, obstetric, and pediatric patients.

Objectives: After reading this chapter and taking this test, you will be able to:

1. Identify expected physiological changes associated with aging.
2. Discuss the emergency care of psychiatric patients.
3. List the physiological changes associated with pregnancy.
4. Describe appropriate emergency care for the pediatric patient.

1. **An 84-year-old presents to the ED reporting a recent onset of lethargy and flu-like symptoms. Which of these assessment findings should you recognize as an expected age-related change?**
   a. long-term memory loss
   b. a widened pulse pressure
   c. hyperactive bowel sounds
   d. decreased pupillary response to light

2. **A family member brings a patient with a history of bipolar disorder who is displaying aggressive and agitated behavior to the ED. When caring for this patient, you should**
   a. avoid making direct eye contact with the patient.
   b. consider the patient violent until proven otherwise.
   c. attempt to calm the patient down by taking his arm in a firm manner.
   d. refrain from engaging the patient in a discussion about physical symptoms.

3. **A patient who is at 32 weeks' gestation is brought to the ED with suspected thoracic injuries following a motor vehicle accident. Which of these ECG changes should you recognize as a finding commonly associated with pregnancy?**
   a. flattened T waves in lead III
   b. elevated ST segments in lead II
   c. the presence of Q waves in lead III
   d. prolonged PR interval in lead II

4. **When assessing the cardiovascular status of a woman who is at 32 weeks' gestation it is a *priority* to notify the physician if this patient has**
   a. a splitting of the first heart sound.
   b. a heart rate of 120 beats per minute.
   c. a central venous pressure of 7 mm Hg.
   d. a decrease in blood pressure when in the supine position.

5. **A 4-year-old patient is brought to the ED by a parent who reports that the child is "not acting right." When performing a triage assessment, you should**
   a. ask a reflective question if the parent appears to be upset.
   b. determine if the parent is overreacting to the child's condition.
   c. recognize that abusive parents often overestimate the seriousness of illness in children.
   d. ask the parent to leave the child's field of vision when performing an initial assessment.

6. **When assessing a child's respiratory status, it is appropriate to**
   a. ask the child to count each respiration.
   b. delay the respiratory assessment if the child is crying.
   c. count the child's respiratory rate before approaching the child.
   d. develop a trusting relationship with the child before performing an assessment.

7. **It is a priority to obtain *immediate* treatment for a pediatric patient who is**
   a. 4 weeks old, is irritable and crying, and has a rectal temperature of 100.6° F.
   b. 9 months old, is pulling at his ears, and is breathing at a rate of 30/minute.
   c. 2 years old, has a vesicular rash on her trunk, and a heart rate of 110 beats per minute.
   d. 4 years old, has a laceration of his left index finger, and a blood pressure of 88/60 mm Hg.

8. **When assessing the vital signs of a pediatric patient, it should be considered an *emergency condition* if a**
   a. 1-week-old has a heart rate of 150, a blood pressure of 60/40 mm Hg, and a respiratory rate of 45/minute.
   b. 1-year-old has a heart rate of 68, a blood pressure of 62/48 mm Hg, and a respiratory rate of 12/minute.
   c. 2-year-old has a heart rate of 92, a blood pressure of 80/52 mm Hg, and a respiratory rate of 28/minute.
   d. 6-year-old has a heart rate of 110, a blood pressure of 100/64 mm Hg, and a respiratory rate of 22/minute.

9. **Which of these immunizations would you expect a 1-month-old infant to have received?**
   a. hepatitis A
   b. hepatitis B
   c. influenza
   d. measles, mumps, rubella (MMR)

10. **Which of these statements is true regarding the 2002 *Suggested Immunization Schedule*?**
   a. The varicella vaccine is initially given to children age 12–15 months.
   b. The first dose of the hepatitis A vaccine must be given by age 4 years.
   c. The activated polio vaccine is given at age 1 month and age 6 months.
   d. The diphtheria, pertussis, tetanus (DPT) immunization is given every 2 months for five doses.

CE Enrollment Form

A Quick Reference to Triage — Part IV — Enhanced Triage: Beyond the Basics

A. Registration Information:

Last name _____ First name _____ MI _____

Address _____

City _____ State _____ Zip _____

Telephone _____ Fax _____ email _____

Registration Deadline: (APRIL 30, 2005)
Contact Hours: 2
Fee: $14.95

B. Test Answers: Darken one for your answer to each question.

	A	B	C	D			A	B	C	D
1.	❏	❏	❏	❏		6.	❏	❏	❏	❏
2.	❏	❏	❏	❏		7.	❏	❏	❏	❏
3.	❏	❏	❏	❏		8.	❏	❏	❏	❏
4.	❏	❏	❏	❏		9.	❏	❏	❏	❏
5.	❏	❏	❏	❏		10.	❏	❏	❏	❏

C. Evaluation*

	A	B
1. Did this CE activity's learning objectives relate to its general purpose?	❏ yes	❏ no
2. Was the home study format an effective way to present the material?	❏ yes	❏ no
3. Was the content relevant to your nursing practice?	❏ yes	❏ no

4. How long did it take you to complete this CE activity?_____hours_____minutes
5. Suggestion for future topics_____

D. Two Easy Ways to Pay:

❏ Check or money order enclosed
(Payable to Lippincott Williams & Wilkins)
Charge my ❏ Mastercard ❏ Visa ❏ American Express
Card #_____ Exp. Date_____
Signature_____

*In accordance with the Iowa Board of Nursing Administrative rules governing grievances, a copy of your evaluation activity may be submitted directly to the Iowa Board of Nursing.

CE Enrollment Form

A Quick Reference to Triage — Part IV — Enhanced Triage: Beyond the Basics

❏ LPN   ❏ RN   ❏ CNS   ❏ NP   ❏ CRNA   ❏ CNM   ❏ other

Job Title _____ Specialty _____

Type of Facility _____

Are you certified?   ❏ yes   ❏ no

Certified by _____

State of License (1) _____ License # _____

State of License (2) _____ License # _____

Social Security # _____

❏ From time to time we make our mailing list available to outside organizations to announce special offers. Please check here if you do not wish us to release your name and address.

CE Test

A Quick Reference to Triage
Part IV – Enhanced Triage: Beyond the Basics

Instructions:

- Read **Part IV** on page **207.**
- Take the test, recording your answers in the test answers section (Section B) of the CE enrollment form. Each question has only one correct answer.
- Complete registration information (Section A) and course evaluation (Section C).
- Mail completed test with registration fee to: Lippincott Williams & Wilkins, CE Depart., 345 Hudson Street, New York, NY 10014.
- Within 3–4 weeks after your CE enrollment form is received, you will be notified of your test results.
- If you pass, you will receive a certificate of earned contact hours and answer key. If you fail, you have the option of taking the test again at no additional cost.
- A passing score for this test is **7** correct answers.
- Need CE STAT? Call 800-833-6525 x331 or x332 for rush service options.
- Questions? Contact Lippincott Williams & Wilkins: (212) 886-1331 or (212) 886-1332.

Registration Deadline: APRIL 30, 2005.

Provider Accreditation:

This Continuing Nursing Education (CNE) activity for **2** contact hours is provided by Lippincott Williams & Wilkins, which is accredited as a provider of continuing education in nursing by the American Nurses Credentialing Center's Commission on Accreditation and by the American Association of Critical-Care Nurses (AACN 9722, CERP Category A). This activity is also provider approved by the California Board of Registered Nursing, Provider Number CEP 11749, for **2** contact hours. LWW is also an approved provider of CNE in Alabama, Florida, and Iowa and holds the following provider numbers: AL #ABNP0114, FL #FBN2454, IA #75. All of its home study activities are classified for Texas nursing continuing education requirements as Type I.

Your certificate is valid in all states. This means that your certificate of earned contact hours is valid no matter where you live.

Payment and Discounts:

- The registration fee for this test is $14.95.
- If you take two or more tests in this book and send in your CE enrollment forms together, you may deduct $1.00 from the price of each test.
- We offer special discounts for as few as six tests and institutional bulk discounts for multiple tests. Call (800) 346-7844, ext. 1286 for more information.

General Purpose: To provide registered professional nurses with an overview of strategies for caring for culturally diverse populations and an update on the Emergency Medical Treatment and Active Labor Act (EMTALA).

Objectives: After reading this chapter and taking this test, you will be able to:

1. Discuss appropriate emergency nursing care when caring for culturally diverse and non-English speaking patients.
2. Describe how to properly care for a patient with a body piercing.
3. Explain the implications of the Emergency Medical Treatment and Active Labor Act (EMTALA) relating to emergency nursing practice.
4. Describe the use of alternative therapies.

1. **Which of these statements is true?**
   a. Those practicing Judaism believe that immunizations are unnecessary.
   b. Haitian immigrants may use rituals of dance and magic for healing purposes.
   c. Individuals of the Baha'i faith believe that life support technology is inappropriate.
   d. Male health care providers should cut the body hair of a male who practices Sikhism.

2. **When caring for a patient in the ED who is a member of a gang, it is important for the nurse to**
   a. avoid leaving medical equipment within the gang member's reach.
   b. recognize that gang members often come to the ED for drugs or violence.
   c. firmly insist that the gang member remove jewelry and head wraps upon arrival.
   d. present herself/himself as the best health care provider this gang member has ever encountered.

3. **A patient presents to the ED with an infected navel body piercing. Appropriate nursing care includes**
   a. applying a wet-to-dry dressing to the site.
   b. obtaining an order to administer the hepatitis A vaccine.
   c. leaving the jewelry in the piercing to allow a channel of drainage.
   d. removing the jewelry and sending it to the lab for culture and sensitivity.

4. **When caring for a patient who presents to the ED with body piercings, you must**
   a. use a ring cutter to remove piercing jewelry.
   b. remove pierced genitalia and navel jewelry prior to applying MAST trousers.
   c. remove jewelry in the nipples before performing external defibrillation.
   d. leave all piercing jewelry in place.

5. **A patient who does not speak English presents to the ED pointing to her head and moaning. When using a translator, it would be important for the triage nurse to**
   a. speak in a loud, monotone voice.
   b. use open-ended questions to obtain information.
   c. verify the translator's ability to interpret appropriately.
   d. face the translator and say, "Ask her to describe her pain."

6. **Which of the following is a violation of the Emergency Medical Treatment and Active Labor Act (EMTALA)?**
   a. Hospital administrators allow an ED to operate short-staffed.
   b. An emergency physician begins assessing a trauma victim in the ambulance of the hospital parking lot.
   c. A pregnant woman insured by Medicaid is transferred to a county hospital while in active labor.
   d. An individual with symptoms of cystitis who is insured by Medicare is made to wait 2 hours before receiving a medical evaluation.

7. **Which of the following herbal medicines has known abortifacient effects?**
   a. St. John's Wort
   b. licorice
   c. soy
   d. horse chestnut

8. **A common cultural practice that leaves the appearance of a cigarette burn may be typically performed in order to treat an individual for**
   a. jaundice.
   b. headache.
   c. tuberculosis.
   d. abdominal pain.

9. **The most commonly practiced cultural remedy involves**
   a. rubbing the edge of a metallic coin or spoon dipped in menthol oil over the symptomatic area.
   b. using orange, lemon, or palm leaves to sweep over the patient's body while reciting prayers to treat illness.
   c. lubricating the skin with mentholated ointment, massaging it, and then pinching the skin over the affected area.
   d. applying suction to a goat horn that has been placed on the patient's forehead and leaving it in place for 15 minutes.

10. **A patient taking prescribed warfarin (Coumadin) should be instructed to avoid which of these herbal medications?**
    a. garlic, ginkgo, and ginseng
    b. acidophilus, peppermint, and soy
    c. echinacea, melatonin, and eucalyptus
    d. flaxseed, glucosamine, and saw palmetto

Glossary

A

Abruptio Placentae — Premature separation of a normal placenta from the uterine wall during the third trimester of pregnancy, resulting in massive hemorrhage

Addiction — Loss of personal control with regard to a chemical or substance

Affect — Moment-to-moment display or expression of human feeling

Aggression — Any verbal, nonverbal, actual, or attempted personal abuse directed toward another person or object

Agnosia — Inability to recognize familiar objects or stimuli

Agoraphobia — Fear and avoidance of being alone, in open spaces, or in an environment from which escape might be difficult. Often presents as a fear of leaving one's own home.

Akathisia — Condition marked by motor restlessness and anxiety

Alzheimer's Disease — Cognitive impairment disorder, with progressive deterioration of function

Anhedonia — Inability to experience pleasure

Anorexia Nervosa — Preoccupation with food and eating combined with intense desire to control food, eating habits, and subsequent body image

Aphasia — Difficulty forming words

Apraxia — Loss of purposeful motor control and movement

Autism — Condition in which thoughts are derived from an internal source, with impaired social interactions and development

B

Battle's Sign — Contusion on the mastoid process of either ear; an indication of a basilar skull fracture

Bipolar Disorder — Mood disorder with variation between manic and depressive episodes

Borderline Personality Disorder — Personality disorder involving impulsive and unpredictable behavior, especially in the areas of behavior, mood, relationships, and self-image

C

Chemical Abuse — Regularly indiscriminate use of a chemical in excess quantities to the extent that a person's psychological, physiologic, and social functioning is impaired

Chemical Dependency — Condition in which the body becomes so accustomed to a drug that body functioning is impaired without it; abruptly stopping the drug causes withdrawal signs and symptoms

Compound Fracture — Opening in the skin over the area of a bone fracture; bone may or may not protrude through the skin

Confabulation — Making up stories or answers to maintain self-esteem when the person does not remember

Conversion — Unconscious transfer of anxiety to a physical symptom that has no organic cause

Crisis — A person's reactive state to a life stressor

D

Delirium — Disturbance in consciousness, accompanied by cognitive changes. Difficulty in mentally focusing, memory, language, orientation, and so on

Delusion — Fixed false belief even when evidence is presented to the contrary

Dementia — Insidious and chronic loss of intellectual function

Depression — Refers to a symptom, a syndrome, a disorder, or an illness that may include overwhelming hopelessness and helplessness that are extremely painful and may be debilitating

Drug Holiday — A brief period of time in which a therapeutic psychiatric medication will be discontinued or tapered to a lower dose. This allows the provider to evaluate the patient's baseline behavior and the possibility of maintaining the patient on a lower dose of medication.

Dysmenorrhea — Painful menstruation

Dyspareunia — Painful intercourse

Dystonia — Usually a side effect of antipsychotic medications, causing muscle spasms of the head, face, neck, and back

Dysuria — Painful or difficult urination

E

Emmenagogue — An agent that promotes menstrual discharge

Estimated Date of Confinement (EDC) — The estimated date of delivery for a pregnant woman

Euphoria — Abnormally exaggerated sense of well-being

Extrapyramidal Side Effects — Abnormal involuntary muscle movements as a result of psychotropic medications. Dystonia, akathisia, and pseudoparkinsonism are reversible; the most serious, tardive dyskinesia, is irreversible.

F

Flat Affect — Absence of facial expression in response to emotion

Flight of Ideas — Rapid movement from one topic of conversation to another—often difficult or impossible for the listener to keep up with

Formication — An abnormal sensation of insect crawling on or in your skin

G

Grandiosity — Exaggerated belief in one's own importance

Gravidity — The number of times a woman is pregnant

H

Hallucination — An alteration in the perception of a body sense when there are no external stimuli present (i.e., smell, vision, touch, hearing, taste)

Hypomania — An elevated mood in which the person maintains connection with reality and experiences no impairment of social, personal, or occupational functioning

I

Ideas of Reference — Unusual or false impressions that outside or external events have a particular personal meaning

Illusion — The misinterpretation of external stimuli (e.g., branches blowing against a roof interpreted as people walking on the roof)

Impulse Disorder — Abrupt and unplanned actions performed in pursuit of instant gratification

L

Labile — Exhibiting rapid changes in emotion

Looseness of Association — Illogical and haphazard thought process

M

Mania — Extreme mental state of mood elevation, with delusions, impaired judgment, and impaired reality orientation

Manic Depression — Disorder of marked alternations in mood

Melancholia — Extreme sadness that inhibits mental and physical activity

Mnemonic Disturbance — Gradually worsening memory loss

Mood — Prevailing emotional tone (e.g., "I feel sad")

N

Narcissism — Intense self-love and self-interest. Normal in children; pathologic in adults when experienced to the same degree as children

Neologism — Self-created words that have meaning only to the person using them

Nontheistic — Traditions in which the holy is conceived of as an impersonal power, a process, a state of being, or an eternal truth capable of transforming human existence

Nuchal Cord — The umbilical cord is wrapped around the neck of the baby during birth

O

Obsession — Preoccupation with persistent, intrusive thoughts that cannot be eliminated by reasoning

P

Paranoia — Strong, irrational opinion unaffected by reality

Parity — The numbers of times a woman has given birth

Perseveration — The repetition of phrases or behavior

Phobia — Strong, irrational fear of an object, activity, or situation

Precipitous Birth — An emergency situation in which birth is imminent, with the desire to push, with crowning occurring. More common in multiparas.

Ptosis — Drooping of the upper eye lid

S

Salter-Harris Fracture — Fracture through the growth plate

Somatization — The expression of psychological stress through physical symptoms

Stridor — A harsh, vibrating sound heard during respiration when there is an airway obstruction

Suppression — Conscious delaying of emotional awareness of a difficult situation or feeling

T

Tardive Dyskinesia — Serious and irreversible side effect of psychotropic medications that involves involuntary muscle movements of the tongue, fingers, toes, neck, trunk, or pelvis

Theistic — Traditions in which the holy is conceived of as God, a group of gods, or spirits personally involved in the life of human beings

W

Word Salad — A mixture of words meaningless to the speaker and listener

Bibliography

ACC/AHA Expert Consensus Document. (1999). Use of sildenafil (Viagra) in patients with cardiovascular disease. *Circulation*, 99, 168–177.

Agency for Toxic Substance and Disease Registry—ATSDR. (2002). (On-line.) http://www.bt.cdc.gov.

American Academy of Pediatrics. (2002). Immunization schedule. (On-line.) http://www.aap.org.

Anderson, R., Kochanek, K., & Murphy, S. (1997). Advance report of final mortality statistics, 1995. *Monthly Vital Statistics Report, 45* (11).

Andrews, M., & Boyle, J. (1995). *Transcultural concepts in nursing care* (2nd ed.). Philadelphia: J.B. Lippincott.

Arnon, S., Schechter, R., Inglesby, R, et al. (2001). Botulinum toxin as a biological weapon. *Journal of the American Medical Association, 285* (8), 1059–1070.

Bartlett, J. (2002). *Pocket book of infectious disease therapy.* Philadelphia: Lippincott Williams & Wilkins.

Beckmann-Murray, R., & Proctor-Zenter, J. (1993). *Nursing assessment and health promotion: Strategies through the life span* (5th ed.). East Norwalk, CT: Appleton & Lange.

Benenson, A. (1995). *Control of communicable diseases manual* (16th ed.). Washington, DC: American Public Health Association.

Blazys, D. (2000). Clinical nurse forum. *Journal of Emergency Nursing, 26* (5), 479–480.

Brewer, J., & Bonalumi, N. (1995). Cultural diversity in the Emergency Department: Health care beliefs and practices among the Pennsylvania Amish. *Journal of Emergency Nursing, 21* (6), 494–497.

Briggs, J. (2001). *Telephone triage protocols for nurses.* Philadelphia: Lippincott Williams & Wilkins.

Cadwell, V. (1995). Christian Science and emergency care: A case of reconciling conflicting beliefs. *Journal of Emergency Nursing, 21* (6), 489–490.

Campbell, R. (1994). *American psychiatric glossary* (7th ed.). Washington, DC: American Psychiatric Press.

Cavanfrisch, N., & Frisch, L. (1998). *Psychiatric mental health nursing* (pp. 352–383). Albany, NY: Delmar Publishers.

Centers for Disease Control and Prevention. (1999). Impaired driving facts. (On-line.) http://www.cdc.gov/ncipc/factsheets/drving.html.

Centers for Disease Control and Prevention. (1998). *Morbidity and Mortality Weekly Report, 47* (8), 161–166.

Cergol, S. (1997). A different reality: Children and mental illness. *Genesee Valley Parents Magazine, 10,* 11–16.

Clemen-Stone, S., Eigsti, D., & McGuire, S. (1995). *Comprehensive community health nursing: Family, aggregate, and community practice* (4th ed.). St. Louis: Mosby-Year Book.

Dart, R. (2000). *The 5-minute toxicology consult.* Philadelphia: Lippincott Williams & Wilkins.

Dennis, D., Inglesby, T., Henderson, D., et al. (2001). Tularemia as a biological weapon: Medical and public health management. *Journal of the American Medical Association, 285* (21), 2763–2773.

DerMarderosian, A. (1999). *A guide to popular natural products.* St. Louis, MO: Facts and Comparisons (a Wolters Kluwer Co.).

Dunbar, A., & Lahn, D. (1998). *Body piercing.* New York: St. Martin's Press.

Edwards, F. (1996). Dermatologic ED presentations: From the mundane to the life-threatening. *Emergency Medicine Reports, 17* (17), 173–179.

Emergency Nurses Association. (1997). *Triage: Meeting the challenge.* Park Ridge, IL: Author.

Frew, S. (2002). COBRA/EMTALA resources: Executive summary. (On-line.) www.medlaw.com.

Frew, S. (1996). COBRA 1996 update. Conference at Niagara Falls Medical Center, Niagara Falls, NY.

Graves, B. (2000). *Tattooing and body piercing: Perspectives on physical health.* Mankato, MN: Capstone Press.

Grossman, V. & McNair, M. (2003). "Gangsta" in the ER! Now what? *American Journal of Nursing, 103* (2).

Hay, W., Groothuis, J., Hayward, A., & Levin, M. (1997). *Current pediatric diagnosis and treatment* (13th ed.). Stamford, CT: Appleton & Lange.

Henderson, D., Inglesby, T., & Bartlett, J. (1999). Smallpox as a biological weapon: Medical and public health management. *Journal of the American Medical Association, 281* (22), 2127–2137.

Hewitt, K. (1997). *Mutilating the body: Identity in blood and ink.* Bowling Green, OH: Bowling Green State University Popular Press.

Hoiting, T., & Harrahil, M. (2000). Cardiac contusion: Two case vignettes. *Journal of Emergency Nursing, 26* (2), 186–187.

Inglesby, T., Henderson, D., Bartlett, J., et al. (1999). Anthrax as a biological weapon: Medical and public health management. *Journal of the American Medical Association, 281* (18), 1735–1745.

Johnson, B.S. (1997). *Adaptation and growth: Psychiatric–mental health nursing* (4th ed.). Philadelphia: Lippincott-Raven.

Joyce, E., & Villanueva, M. (1996). *Say it in Spanish.* Philadelphia: W.B. Saunders.

Kendrick, K., Baxi, S., & Smith, R. (2000). Usefulness of the modified 0–10 Borg scale in assessing the degree of dyspnea in patients with COPD and asthma. *Journal of Emergency Nursing, 26* (3), 216–222.

Lippincott manual of nursing practice (6th ed.). (1996). Philadelphia: J.B. Lippincott.

McFarlane, J., Greenberg, L., Weltge, A., & Watson, M. (1995). Identification of abuse in emergency departments: Effectiveness of a two-question screening tool. *Journal of Emergency Nursing, 21* (5), 391–394.

McGregor, N., & Barnet, V. (2002). Personal communication.

Mercury, M. (2000). *The alchemy of body modification: Pagan fleshworks*. Rochester, VT: Park Press.

Miller, J. (1997). *The body art book*. New York: The Berkley Publishing Group.

Molczan, K. (2001). Triaging orthopedic injuries. *Journal of Emergency Nursing, 27* (3), 297–300.

Murphy, K. (1997). *Pediatric triage guidelines*. St. Louis: Mosby-Year Book.

Mutch, P., & Grossman, V. (2001). A 22-year-old woman with exquisite burning pain 4 weeks after an ankle sprain. *Journal of Emergency Nursing, 27* (3), 234–237.

National Center for Injury Prevention and Control. (2002). Suicide in the United States: Suicide prevention fact sheet. (On-line.) http://www.cdc.gov/ncipc/factsheets/suifacts.htm.

National Council on Alcoholism and Drug Dependence. (2000). Alcoholism and alcohol-related problems. (On-line.) http://www.ncass.org/facts/problems.html.

National Institute of General Medical Sciences. (2001). Trauma, burn, shock, and injury: Facts and figures. (On-line.) http://www.nigms.nih.gov/news/facts/traumaburnfactsfigure.

National Institute of Health. (1995). *Heart attacks*. No. 95-2645. Rockville, MD: U.S. Department of Health and Human Services.

National Institute on Alcohol Abuse and Alcoholism. (1997). *Alcohol alert: Alcohol-related impairment*. No. 38. Rockville, MD: U.S. Department of Health and Human Services.

National Institute on Alcohol Abuse and Alcoholism. (1994). *Alcohol alert: Alcohol-related impairment*. No. 25 PH 351. Rockville, MD: U.S. Department of Health and Human Services.

Nettina, S. (1997). *Lippincott's pocket manual of nursing practice*. Philadelphia: Lippincott-Raven.

Rebmann, T. (2001). What infection control practitioners need to know to be prepared for a bioterrorism attack. *Infection Control Today, 5* (12), 24–27.

RNCEUS.COM. (2002). Biochemical terrorism: An emergency room resource. (On-line.) http://www.rnceus.com.

Roberts, C. (1997). Focus on thrombolytic therapy for acute ischemic stroke. *Heartbeat: A Cardiac Nursing Newsletter, 7* (2), 1–11.

Roper, M. (1996). Back to basics: Assessing orthostatic vital signs. *American Journal of Nursing, 96* (8), 43–46.

Rosen, P., Barkin, R., Hayden, R., Schaider, J., & Wolfe, R. (1999). *The 5-minute emergency medicine consult*. Philadelphia: Lippincott Williams & Wilkins.

Sachs, S. (1997). *Street gang awareness*. Minneapolis, MN: Fairview Press.

Schmitt, B. (2000). *Pediatric telephone protocols*. Philadelphia: Lippincott Williams & Wilkins.

Sinclair, C. (1996). *Handbook of obstetrical emergencies*. Philadelphia: W.B. Saunders.

Thompson, D.A. (2001). *Adult telephone triage algorithms, 185 Topics*. Chicago, IL.

Valentine, B. (2000). *Gangs and their tattoos: Identifying gang-bangers on the street and in prison*. Boulder, CO: Paladin Press.

Varcarolis, E. (1998). *Foundations of psychiatric mental health nursing* (3rd ed.). Philadelphia: W.B. Saunders.

Wilkinson, B. (1998). *Coping with the dangers of tattooing, body piercing, and branding*. New York: The Rosen Publishing Group, Inc.

Wolbert-Burgess, A. (1997). *Psychiatric nursing: Promoting mental health*. Stamford, CT: Appleton & Lange.

Zavotsky, K., Sapienza, J., & Wood, D. (2001). Nursing implications for ED care of patients who have received heart transplants. *Journal of Emergency Nursing, 27* (1), 33–39.

INDEX

Note: Page numbers followed by f,t, and b indicate figures, tables, and boxed material, respectively.